Tell Me Where It Hurts

HOW TO DECIPHER YOUR CHILD'S EMOTIONAL ACHES AND PHYSICAL PAINS

JONATHAN A. SLATER, M.D.,
AND MARK L. FUERST

Adams Media Corporation
Avon, Massachusetts

Dedication

I dedicate this book to my family: to my parents, Sonny and Dena, whose love and belief in me has been the foundation upon which my life rests; to my wife, Lori, my greatest ally and partner, whose love, support, and understanding have allowed me to pursue my dreams; to my two sisters, Elizabeth and Marjorie, who are always there for me; and to my four children, Carly, Hannah, Zach, and Logan, whose love provides me with inspiration that warms my heart and carries me through each day.

—JS

I also dedicate this book to my family: my parents, Joel and Peppy; my wife, Margie; my two children, Ben and Sarah; and my brother Jeff and his family—for their love and support through this project, and in life.

—MF

Published by
Adams Media Corporation
57 Littlefield Street, Avon, MA 02322 U.S.A.
www.adamsmedia.com

ISBN: 1-58062-621-1

Printed in Canada.

J I H G F E D C B A

Library of Congress Cataloging-in-Publication Data
Slater, Jonathan A., M.D.
Tell me where it hurts: how to decipher your child's emotional aches and physical pains / by Jonathan A. Slater and Mark L. Fuerst.
p. cm.   Includes bibliographical references and index.
ISBN 1-58062-621-1
1. Pediatrics–Psychosomatic aspects. I. Fuerst, Mark L. II. Title.
RJ47.5 .S58 2002
618.92'008–dc21

2002008505

This publication is designed to provide accurate and authoritative information with regard to the subject matter covered. It is sold with the understanding that the publisher is not engaged in rendering legal, accounting, or other professional advice. If legal advice or other expert assistance is required, the services of a competent professional person should be sought.
—From a *Declaration of Principles* jointly adopted by a Committee of the American Bar Association and a Committee of Publishers and Associations

Cover image by Rolf Bruderer/Corbis Stockmarket

This book is available at quantity discounts for bulk purchases.
For information call 1-800-872-5627.

Table of Contents

Part I
What Your Child Isn't Telling You About Aches and Pains

Part II
Finding Out What's Going On

Part III
Helping Your Child Feel Better

Foreword

by Clarice J. Kestenbaum, M.D.

Professor of Clinical Psychiatry/Director of Training,
Child and Adolescent Psychiatry at Columbia University;
Immediate Past President, American Academy of Child and Adolescent Psychiatry

RICE PUDDING
By A.A. Milne

What is the matter with Mary Jane?
She's crying with all her might and main,
And she won't eat her dinner-rice pudding again—
What is the matter with Mary Jane?

What is the matter with Mary Jane?
I've promised her dolls and a daisy-chain,
And a book about animals—all in vain—
What is the matter with Mary Jane?

What is the matter with Many Jane?
She's perfectly well, and she hasn't a pain,
But look at her, now she's beginning again!—
What is the matter with Mary Jane?

What is the matter with Mary Jane?
I've promised her sweets and a ride in the train,
And I've begged her to stop for a bit and explain—
What is the matter with Mary Jane?

What is the matter with Mary Jane?
She's perfectly well and she hasn't a pain.
And it's lovely rice pudding for dinner again!—
What is the matter with Mary Jane?

A.A. Milne, creator of Winnie-the-Pooh, who wrote these lines almost eighty years ago, got it right. What is the matter with Mary Jane and Billie and Max and the thousands of other children who appear in our offices each year? Are their problems emotional, physical, or a combination of both?

Dr. Slater answers this question as only a "compleat physician" can: as a doctor, child psychiatrist, psychoanalyst, scholar, father, and humanist.

His approach to discovering the origin of a problem is to listen to the patient and try to understand how that person's mind/body is at play. His book is a rich compilation of case studies and examples, including the most up-to-date findings on neurology, autoimmune disease, psychiatric disorders, learning disabilities, and evidence-based treatment approaches.

Research over recent decades has yielded startling findings on the effectiveness of mind/body therapy. We now have a growing body of data on the power of the mind to temper—if not overcome—physical hardship, as well as a deepening knowledge of the biological foundations of many psychiatric disorders. The inescapable conclusion is that the most effective therapy for any malaise is that which combines a variety of mental health treatments.

Dr. Slater presents compelling evidence that the brain can be altered by experience. In fact, a parent's nurturing style can actually alter a child's nature or innate biology.

Dr. Slater offers readers a wealth of material, including a mood chart, checklists, questionnaires, and helpful practical suggestions that will take communication between parent and child to a whole new level.

Tell Me Where It Hurts is an invaluable resource and a superb guide for the perplexed parent, pediatrician, mental health professional, and patient. Dr. Slater clarifies age-old misconceptions about mental illness and ways to heal, with sensitivity, profound insight, and prose that is at once lucid and accessible.

My seven-year-old daughter Hannah began complaining about a stomachache on the day I was to leave on a business trip. As I got her ready for bed, she stared over at her pet cockatiel Flutter and began talking about the first cockatiel we had bought, Buttercup, which had died one week after we took it home. Hannah would sometimes lament that she had never taken a picture of herself with Buttercup. When her stomach began to hurt more, I took the timing as a cue that maybe her physical and emotional feelings also had to do with my going away.

"Sweetie, do you think that maybe you're feeling bad and thinking about Buttercup because you're going to miss me?" I asked. Hannah melted into my arms and cried softly, nodding her head. We arranged times that I would call her while I was gone, and talked about the hat that she wanted me to bring back for her. When I kissed her good-bye, her tummy was feeling better.

Translation: "My tummy hurts because I'm going to miss my Daddy."

Preface

Tell Me Where It Hurts takes a new approach to psychosomatic illnesses, translating the latest in biochemical and behavioral research into practical information for today's parents. Parents learn how the mind interacts with the body, how to evaluate their child's physical symptoms and when symptoms may be masking emotional difficulties, and how to reduce the stresses associated with illnesses.

Readers will also learn how to recognize when physical symptoms might be part of a syndrome with emotional problems. Chronic stomachaches, headaches, and muscle and joint pain may signal an anxiety disorder or depression. As many as 30 percent of children report frequent headaches, up to 25 percent have recurrent abdominal pain, and some 20 percent complain of muscle and joint pains, according to recent research. These symptoms may also indicate the beginning of long-term problems— up to half of all children with recurrent stomachaches continue to suffer them as adults.

These and other symptoms can be a source of significant upset within the family, and can affect the child's social and academic functioning. The coping tools Dr. Slater teaches his patients and their parents can come into play *before* a child gets sick. All parents can learn the simple techniques presented in this book and prevent many of the problems that lead 100 million children to see a pediatrician each year.

Children often say things in subtle, at times vague, or even misleading ways. Perhaps we should call this "lost language" of childhood "kidspeak"—

the way children signal what they have to say, sometimes more often with their bodies and their behavior than their words. This book helps parents of children of all ages and developmental levels go into the inner workings of a child's mind, see childhood problems in a different way, and learn techniques to decipher the often-complicated signals children use instead of language to communicate.

A better understanding of these signals can also help parents interpret more complex physical symptoms and emotional states. A parent takes a child to the doctor to help decipher the underlying cause of physical symptoms. The doctor does an examination, and may run some tests, to diagnose what the particular symptoms represent, or translate what the child's body is trying to say. Similarly, a psychiatrist or psychologist looks at a set of symptoms or behaviors, and often without the benefit of an actual test, interprets the meaning behind the symptoms.

Tell Me Where It Hurts teaches parents how to develop this type of skilled observation. When children don't feel well, they often don't tell their parents about it. When they do, children often express their feelings in subtle ways. In general, younger children especially are not that aware of underlying emotional issues. So when they complain of physical pains, they may not realize that underlying feelings may be surfacing in a "physical" way. Children may also lack the capacity to describe their feelings the way adults do. Young children, in particular, often lack the language skills or the ability to step outside themselves and look at the way they feel.

It becomes the parent's job to interpret these signals. With an infant, a parent learns, and is actually taught by the baby, to know which type of cry is a wet-diaper cry, as opposed to a cry of hunger, fatigue, or pain. Parents can also learn how to decode the more complex emotional and physical signals of older children. In translating the signals, by being more tuned in to the actual problem at hand, they can act more empathically and effectively.

Parents will become familiar with the common ways children try to say things while not really saying them. For example, depressed children and young adolescents may have difficulty in describing their emotions or moods. They may not complain about how bad they feel, and instead may act moody and cranky. Parents and teachers may not recognize this behavior as a sign of depression. *Tell Me Where It Hurts* simplifies and categorizes the different types of reactions children may have to both physical and emotional illnesses and the typical ways they communicate their distress through behavior. These explanations help parents to become better readers of the pages of the book of childhood.

Each of the book's anecdotes contains the message a child gave to describe what was wrong, followed immediately by a "translation" of what might really be on the child's mind. Parents can learn to use these models to become more keenly aware of their children's underlying messages when they are sick. Each chapter ends with an Action Plan and Action Points summarizing the material presented and suggesting what to do with the information, for example, how to get help, what to do at home, or when to go to the doctor.

Tell Me Where It Hurts goes behind the physical, looking at all areas, or "domains," of your child's or adolescent's life and the various challenges he or she faces, ranging from emotional disorders and learning disabilities to violence and the Internet. The domains examined include: your child's feelings; how your child thinks and speaks; how your child functions and behaves; how your child relates to family members, friends, teachers, coaches, or mentors; your child's environment (home, school, athletic teams); and how your child relates to himself or herself and how the domains relate to each other.

This book reviews how you as a parent can help your child by using, among other things, stress reduction, sports and other activities, traditional medicine, and alternative medicine. The goal is to help you understand and communicate with your child, and find the best ways to help your child grow into a happy, confident adult.

Acknowledgments

We would like to thank our agent Faith Hamlin for her persistence and support throughout the project, and the staff at Adams Media for helping to put it all together.

Many people helped us in the long process of making this book a reality. We would like to acknowledge writer-friends Janice Tanne for hooking us up and Judith Horstman for coming up with a great title, as well as the ASJA Brooklyn Bag Lunch group for brainstorming and encouragement.

Jon would also like to especially acknowledge Shihan Jim Chillemi, for his ever-present spiritual support and positive energy, which shapes the lives of so many people fortunate enough to know him. He would also like to acknowledge his mother, Dena Slater, for her tremendous help editing the manuscript, which was a labor of love.

He would also like to thank Clarice Kestenbaum, M.D., for being a major guiding force in his professional life, a "second mother," and a model of what a child psychiatrist should be. Lastly, he would like to express gratitude to Candy Erickson, for reviewing and editing portions of the manuscript, and for being such an important mentor throughout the years.

PART I

What Your Child Isn't

Telling You About

Aches and Pains

CHAPTER 1

My Child Doesn't Talk to Me

"How was school today?"
"Good."
"What'd you do?"
"Nothing."

Sound familiar? Sometimes it's tough to get children to talk about their day, and even the most persistent parent may give up after the third or fourth one- or two-word answer. Through a parent's eyes, the child may seem just not interested or even bothered by the same old daily questions.

Readers might be surprised to find out what it's like from the child's perspective, which is the purpose of this chapter. The central premise is that children do communicate with parents, who just have to become better listeners. Parents must avoid imposing adult points of view and agendas on their children. With my guidelines, parents can get a sense of what goes on in their child's life, which often entails spending time away from home in school, with friends, or with the parents of friends.

Between the Lines

When eight-year-old Sophia arrives home from second grade, the only thing on her mind is getting a snack and finding a play date for those precious hours before dinner. As she steps off the bus, school becomes a distant memory. "Parents are weird. They tell each other all about their day over dinner. How boring!" she tells me.

Sophia's best time to talk is right before bed, when she just "feels like it," or when she's traveling in the car and the hypnotic motion lends itself to her most curious thoughts. "Sometimes I feel like my parents aren't ready to talk to me about things, like the time I asked them, when we were on the way to summer vacation, how babies were made," she says.

Translation: "When my parents ask me about school, it's annoying, as if they have to know the answers to their questions at a time that's best for them. A lot of times I'd rather not say how I feel, and wish they could just tell what's on my mind."

Two basic things children want from their parents are to be listened to and to be understood. The keys to talking to children are listening, timing, and being receptive to their questions, whenever and wherever they occur, as well as reading signals and translating behavior. Many parents do this unconsciously in familiar situations. For example, they may know that the late-afternoon bewitching hour for young children, when their crankiness is predictable, has to do with fatigue and hunger, not necessarily true irritation.

Effective parents need to listen beyond the sniffles of childhood. Important nonverbal signals, such as body posture, eye contact, and tone of voice, can help parents "read" what their children are really saying. Interpreting physical signals, such as complaints of headaches or joint or abdominal pains, become all the more important because most children don't spontaneously say what's on their minds. Lots of times, however, the door is open and they are just waiting for a parent to approach them.

A parent needs to be a detective, gleaning clues from the behavior and language of the child, and from conversations with other parents and teachers. Like a detective, you may ask direct questions and receive evasive answers. Your best tools are observation, logical thinking, intuition, and luck.

What's on a Child's Mind

Sometimes, I'll spend fifteen or twenty minutes with a child, meet with the child's parents, and recount my impressions of what's on the child's mind. "You got all that?!" the parents may ask incredulously, and then want to know how I did it. The answer lies in straightforward, simple techniques to help parents talk to children:

- Meet the child on his or her own level. If a toddler cries over a boo-boo, hold, comfort, and rock him or her. Once he or she calms down, then you can ask what happened.
- Go on a fishing expedition—throw out a line (a leading question) and see if the child will nibble. If not, don't persist. Never pressure a child to talk about something. It won't work, and will probably make the child more resistant.
- If a child shows what's on her or his mind through a subtle response, comment, or association, that's the time to ask a more direct question about what's going on.
- Play a game as you talk. With younger children, in particular, you can often talk about a subject without ever talking directly about it, using a storytelling game or a squiggle art game invented by D. H. Winnicott, a British pediatrician and psychoanalyst.

Here's an example of how I use squiggle art, a technique described by Winnicott, to help a child open up. Lauren, an exquisitely shy seven-year-old girl, loved to draw pictures of fish. When I drew a squiggle on paper, she turned it into a fish. At my suggestion, she made up a story about the fish. "The fish is lonely because she has no friends," Lauren said. I asked if I could add something to her picture, and when she said I could, I drew squiggles of some other fish playing in another part of the pond. I asked her if her fish could swim over and say hello. "She couldn't because she doesn't know what to say, and she's afraid the other fish would say, 'No.' And maybe her scales aren't as pretty as the others," Lauren said. I rehearsed ways that her fish could join the others, giving her specific lines, and I became the other fish, saying (what I knew to be true from her mother) that the other fish actually liked her and wondered why she wouldn't play with them. I told Lauren, that maybe she was unsure about how her scales looked, but to the other fish, I bet they looked just fine.

Lauren and I met several times and played art games. Along with encouragement from her mother to have play dates, and my suggestion that her teacher facilitate social contact at school, Lauren began to approach other children more comfortably. Lauren and I never spoke directly about her shyness; it was all done indirectly through play.

Translation: "I know exactly what you're talking about. Just don't talk to me directly because it makes me too nervous."

Time Is on My Side

Children think about time differently from adults. Children live in the present and have a poor memory of even the recent past. They don't have a good capacity to reflect on the day's events and what they were feeling. To help your detective work, I suggest that you take the child back in time to a particular place, and then ask questions about it. For example, if you want to really find out what happened in school, you might say to your child, "Make believe you just got to school. Who are you sitting next to? What kind of work are you doing?" Or ask, "When you got to the cafeteria for lunch, who did you eat with? What did you talk about?" If you know something about your child's school day, by all means use it. Ask, "What did you do in gym class today?" Let the answers guide your next set of questions. You'll be amazed how much more information you can glean.

Write It Down

There's tremendous value in a child's keeping a daily journal or diary. This activity can help provide a sense of reflection and encourage autonomy, as well as being fun for school-age children and adolescents. Journal writing challenges children to develop a more narrative sense of themselves and not to just live in the moment.

Children's journals are also a useful tool to rate the pain of chronic problems and to identify regular patterns, say, headaches before quizzes or stomachaches on Mondays. I have children with mood problems who are taking medications use journals to record their feelings. When they note their moods on a scale of zero to three it gives them a sense of how things change by the days of the week or the seasons. You may want to use the following Monthly Mood Chart with your child to help you identify such patterns.

Monthly Mood Chart

Rate each item below daily for one month, using 0 = None, 1 = Mild, 2 = Moderate, and 3 = Severe.

	1	2	3	4	5	6	7	8	9	10	11	12	13	14	15	16	17	18	19	20	21	22	23	24	25	26	27	28	29	30
Depressed mood																														
Anxiety																														
Irritability																														
Sleep problems																														
Physical Symptoms																														
Abdominal pain																														
Nausea																														
Diarrhea																														
Headaches																														
Joint pains																														
Fatigue																														
Dizziness																														
Vomiting																														

Daily notes (stresses, events):

Action Plan

Practice the following techniques and see what works best for you to help your child open up. It may take some time for you to get the hang of it. Once you start listening and understanding better, you'll learn more about your child's life because your child will begin to share things more spontaneously with you, without your having to ask.

Make time to attend more of your child's school, social, and athletic activities. Even just taking time to drop off and pick up your child can mean a lot. You'd be surprised what can come out during a car ride. The motion of the road often has a calming effect that allows your child's thoughts to wander and makes it easier to open up emotionally.

Play games with your children, such as board games or tabletop games, or catch or kick a ball. These activities also provide an opportunity to interact with your child and help your child feel comfortable and talk about other things in a more relaxed environment.

Do you know how to play with your child? Take some time to ask yourself how you and your child play together. How much of what you do is what your child chooses? How much is your just taking him or her places? Ask your child what he or she wants to do, and make time to do it.

Draw pictures, write stories, or build things with your child. Read a story to your child, or have the child read to you. Talk about what you've drawn or read or done. Act the same way as the characters in the story, and ask your child how he or she felt while you were reading the story. Ask, "What do you think was the point of story?" You can also make television watching more active by asking what the characters are feeling. You'll gain an increased understanding of how your child feels and thinks using these techniques.

Buy your child a book with blank pages to write her or his private thoughts in. Promise the child you won't read it, and keep that promise—*don't read it.*

Getting a child to talk to you is something you have to work on. Once you gain the child's trust and respect the child's wishes, then you'll get much more information.

Action Points

1. Listen to your child to understand him or her better.
2. Hang out with your child in relaxing situations to help feelings and thoughts flow freely.
3. Talk about the feelings of the characters in books you read or those you see on television.
4. Buy your child a diary to write in and respect his or her privacy.

CHAPTER 2

The Mind and the Body—
It's Not All in Your Head

*T*hirteen-year-old Teddy was referred to me by his pediatrician after weeks of tummy pain and many missed school days. His parents had tried everything from laxatives to a better diet to heating pads. Teddy's belly has been poked and prodded during several pediatrician visits, his stool cultured, his blood tested, and his abdomen x-rayed. All the results were negative. What's more, Teddy began to get headaches. He began playing less with his friends, looked unhappy, and felt physically worse in the morning when he "tried" to go to school. His parents, exasperated with him, felt he was faking the pain because he didn't want to go to school.

After careful examination, I found that Teddy was quite sad, had trouble sleeping and concentrating, was not enjoying anything, had become isolated from his friends, had no energy, and even was thinking about death. I diagnosed Teddy with clinical depression, which was not surprising since both of his parents' families had a history of depression. I treated Teddy with cognitive behavioral psychotherapy, and taught him some relaxation techniques to use when the pain struck. Given the fact that progress was slow after four weeks, I also suggested that Teddy start taking one of the newer antidepressants. Within a few weeks, he felt less tummy and headache pain, and felt good enough to go to school again. I worked with his school to reduce his workload while he recovered. He said that his body no longer felt "out of whack." After several months, I took Teddy off the medicine, and he did fine; all of his systems were back "on line."

Translation: "I really don't feel well and I don't know why. I'm upset because my parents don't believe me, and I'm sick of all the doctors and tests. I'm bummed out to the point where I don't feel like hanging out with my friends."

This chapter synthesizes recent neurological, gastrointestinal, anxiety, and depression research into easy-to-follow steps for parents. This research can help parents become oriented toward the world beyond their child's physical complaints. Parents who evaluate symptoms and interpret body language can make decisions about their children's care from both medical and psychological perspectives. Heightening parents' awareness of the mind-body connection can help them identify and treat some physical symptoms early, and prevent other problems from becoming chronic.

Nature Equals Nurture

As an infant, one of my daughters became attached to her mother from the age of one year on. She found it hard to be out of her mother's sight and got nervous when she played with new toys or went into a new setting. My wife and I initially disagreed about what to do. She suggested that since my daughter might have a more anxious temperament, that we shouldn't stress her at such a young age, and should keep her home. On the other hand, I'm a firm believer that experience can shape personality. So we found a nurturing preschool for my daughter at age two. Although the separation from her mother was difficult at first, by the middle of the year she became more comfortable being away from her mother and more flexible in enjoying new experiences.

Translation: "I'm cranky because it's my way of saying I'm scared. Something bad might happen to me without my Mommy there to protect me."

One of the central tenets of modern-day neurobiology is that the brain can be altered by experience. Studies using specialized imaging techniques to record changes in the brain dramatize how changing someone's feelings through successful behavior and interpersonal psychotherapy actually change the brain. This knowledge puts enormous power into parents' hands.

While biology determines most everything when it comes to illness, a parent's nurturing style can alter a child's nature or innate biology. Harvard University psychologist Jerome Kagan and his colleagues have found that three-fourths of kids who are behaviorally inhibited, meaning that they become upset when presented with novel stimuli early in infancy, remain temperamentally anxious as they grow up. But that means that one-fourth do not. When explaining why those children are unaffected researchers credit a calming parenting approach and positive social experiences.

This temperamental predisposition in a child must be "actualized," or brought out, the researchers say. The way parents behave toward a child can often affect a child's developing temperament. Aggressive behavior by an older brother or sister, a long stretch in the hospital, or household squabbling may intensify a child's inability to handle stress. With a parent's encouragement and guidance, these children can learn how to deal with stressful situations without expressing their anxiety.

The implication of research by Nobel Prize winner Eric Kandel of Columbia University is that experience can alter gene expression. If one takes somewhat of a leap of faith—one that I believe is justified—parents' behavior may be able to alter their children's brain physiology. A calm parenting style may override the "predetermined" way that a child manifests anxious symptoms. Even if a child is naturally prone to being anxious, a nurturing parent can remain calm and help a child repeatedly master anxious experiences, as opposed to "enabling" a child to anxiously avoid these experiences. In this way, the child's brain may actually be changed! Over time, this approach may help the child feel more comfortable with new experiences.

Immune to Stress

The brain and the immune system influence each other. Stress, for example, can affect immune function, and your immune status can affect behavior. Studies show that children can use self-hypnosis, relaxation, and imagery techniques to boost their immune systems and actually decrease the incidence of upper-respiratory infections.

Recognizing the implications of stress and immunity can help parents make their children healthier. For example, pediatrician Karen Olness, M.D., from Case Western Reserve University (in the book *Hypnosis and Hypnotherapy with Children*, written with Daniel P. Kohen, M.D.), tells how she conditioned an eleven-year-old girl who had problems with hives when she skated competitively. The young skater imagined a "joystick" in her mind that could turn off the cells in her skin that secreted the histamine that caused the immune response. The hives stopped, and she did not have to take antihistamines, which would have limited her ability to skate competitively.

The Physical (Sometimes) Equals the Emotional

More and more medical research is linking physical and emotional symptoms. Joseph Levy, M.D., a pediatric gastroenterologist at New York–Presbyterian, is conducting research to measure the electrical activity of the stomach to find out what may be causing recurrent abdominal pain. Researchers at the National Institutes of Health have proven that the brains of anxious children are different than those of normal children. Other studies report that children with disruptive behavior disorders have higher rates of obesity and elevated blood pressure, and that anxious girls do not grow as tall as expected.

The Brain, Behavior, and Stress

New research relates childhood behavior to brain, immune, and endocrine functioning. In particular, the stress hormone cortisol has been linked to childhood disease and brain development. The biological consequences of stress have been demonstrated in animal studies of parents that were stressed during pregnancy and their offspring that were stressed in infancy, just when brain development naturally begins. Several studies show that high levels of cortisol lead to a lower resistance to infection among children. Other research shows the incidence of childhood illness is related to the interaction of stress and arterial pressure reactivity, which measures the flexibility of arteries.

Children who have just started kindergarten, a stressful time for them, show higher cortisol levels in their saliva and a lower immune response.

Studies of children with behavior problems reveal declines in immune function, and others show that depressed immune function is correlated with behavioral problems. Behavior is linked to immune function and stress by cortisol's effects on the immune system. A few studies have looked at which immune changes go along with minor stresses. Others have looked at large changes. The significance of these studies is that researchers are now using biological parameters to show the effects of stress on children's behavior. These findings shed a different light on physical problems—the children in these studies are not just acting out and being manipulative. Their behavior has biological underpinnings that are mediated by stress hormones.

Some children's brains are more susceptible to stressful events. Studies of brain wave patterns show individual differences in how children respond immunologically to stress. Researchers have found changes in white blood cell counts associated with stressful life events among children who have specific brain wave patterns. These children perceive stress as more adverse and, as a result, have lower immune function.

Behavior also has been associated with how the heart reacts. One study by University of California at Irvine psychologist J. Quas shows that when three- to six-year-olds were asked to complete a challenging task, as their heart rates increased, their facial expressions became more exaggerated, particularly among girls. The implication of this research is, again, that biology and behavioral emotional systems are coupled.

Social Support

Psychiatric interventions for adults with malignant melanoma and breast cancer have shown that group therapy is associated with positive changes in immune function

These findings underscore the effects of stress on immune function. Greater social support may lead to improved survival in certain types of cancer. We can do things that involve emotional, social interventions to affect biology and the outcome of disease. This knowledge should empower parents in dealing with their children. Look carefully for stress in your child and at how much emotional support you provide. You may be able to change some biological parameters, such as immune function, susceptibility to disease, and even heart function, with more support.

Several major studies from Columbia University researchers show how heart rate variability, a measure of how flexible the beating of the heart is, relates to depression and anxiety. A strong predictor of death following a heart attack is reduced heart rate variability. Hostile people who are also depressed and anxious have low heart rate variability, and may be at increased risk of dying of heart rhythm problems. After a heart attack, depressed people have higher mortality rates. Men with phobic anxiety also have a higher rate of dying of heart disease. Depression, anxiety, hostility, and anger all affect heart function.

Parents want to be able to recognize depression, anxiety, hostility, and anger in their children, and then to deal with it. We now know these psychological problems have profound biological consequences in adults, which is yet another link between emotion and biology. Minimizing these problems early on may help prevent the connection to heart disease later in life.

Cortisol and Sleep

Depressed adolescents often have a hard time falling asleep, and this has been linked to higher cortisol levels. A child who doesn't get enough sleep and is fatigued during the day will likely have problems modulating his or her emotions. In fact, a sleep-deprived child can present a picture that looks like attention deficit hyperactivity disorder. But sleep problems may be an early sign of depression among adolescence.

Now, the idea is not for parents to start having fancy tests to measure their teens' cortisol levels, which is how biological connections can get misused. Adolescents' sleep patterns normally change with age. Between ages ten and thirteen, children's sleep time decreases, and teens tend to spend more time in bed on weekends compared to weekdays. Teens may have problems falling asleep because they are up later on weekends, despite their need for more sleep as they go through puberty. So a sleep problem by itself is not enough to say an adolescent is depressed.

Yet, insomnia may be an early sign of depression, and depression is correlated with cortisol abnormalities. Parents need to find out what is keeping their teen up. Is your child staring at the ceiling in bed, staying up doing homework, or going out late with friends? See what is going on during the week and put it into context. Go over the signs and symptoms of depression in Chapter 6. Talk with your teen about why he or she is having trouble sleeping. Try to present information about good sleep hygiene to help your teen decide what's good for him or her. If your child continues to have sleep problems, ask your pediatrician for help and, if need be, see a mental health professional.

Imaging Studies

New imaging studies provide more evidence of the correlation between emotional problems and brain changes. These positron emission tomography (PET) scan studies show a relationship between anorexia and greater stimulation in different parts of the brain, between posttraumatic stress disorder and greater regional differences in blood flow in certain parts of the brain, and brain changes among children who have been sexually abused. Migraine sufferers process signals to the vision center in the brain more rapidly than people who don't have migraines, and therefore appear to be oversensitive to visual stimuli. Other researchers are looking at how different parts of the brain are activated when subjects look at different types of objects. Mapping the circuitry in the brain could help psychiatrists diagnose mental illnesses, and possibly lead to new therapies.

The Second Brain

Tim, a well-adjusted sixteen-year-old, had a long history of stomachaches and headaches, which seem to persist following viral infections. Over the years, he had multiple diagnostic procedures, including both upper and lower gastrointestinal series, CAT scans, and endoscopies. More alarming, he had surgery to remove what was a normal appendix. Tim had been out of school and essentially homebound for months when he was referred to me.

I found it striking that Tim seemed to be emotionally stable and denied feeling anxious or depressed. After reviewing his histories of multiple visits to specialists, it was clear that we had to try a different approach, especially since serious physical illnesses had been ruled out. I taught Tim some self-hypnosis exercises and put him on a program of progressive muscle relaxation and stress reduction. He also had the school psychologist do some testing, which found a subtle learning disability that had not been picked up before. I suggested that the school lighten his academic load and get him a tutor. Tim and I practiced some coping strategies for stressful situations. I put him on a low dose of a selective serotonin reuptake inhibitor (SSRI), one of the newer antidepressants. Using these medications may seem drastic, but most of these patients have been on multiple medications, have had invasive procedures, repeated tests, and serious impairment in how they function. In these situations, my colleagues and I have had some success using these medications for recurrent abdominal pain not caused by a treatable gastrointestinal condition, or in conjunction with other medicines that are being used to treat symptoms such as pain and constipation.

Within several weeks, Tim was well on the road to full recovery. He was about to begin "triple-sessions" (three practices in one day) for his high school football team. He said that the abdominal pain was gone and that he could ignore his headaches with the strategies he had learned.

Translation: "I don't feel well and nothing seems to help me get better. I don't trust my body anymore. I was having some trouble in school before, and now I've missed so much school, I'll never catch up, so why bother going."

Exciting new revelations about an independently functioning neural system in the gastrointestinal tract known as the "second brain," which Columbia University's Michael Gershon, M.D., outlines in his book of the same name, have helped revolutionize thinking about how the gastrointestinal tract operates. A girl who is taking one of the newer SSRI antidepressants, which alter how the body uses serotonin, to treat depression may find that her recurrent stomachaches ease as well. The same treatment for serotonin levels in her brain may work on the serotonin in her gut, which is second only to the brain in level of serotonin.

Gershon's groundbreaking work clearly demonstrates that the gut actually has a brain of its own. In many ways, the second brain in the gut normally works independently of the brain, as well as in concert with the brain in the head. The familiar term "nervous stomach" points to an interaction between the central nervous system, found throughout the body, and the enteric nervous system, the digestive control center or so-called "second brain" found only in the gut.

What's more, new studies indicate that a serotonin dysfunction may be a common abnormality for children who are depressed, anxious, aggressive, or who suffer from recurrent headaches. Serotonin appears to affect multiple organs and influence multiple diseases.

The Interaction of Physical and Emotional Symptoms

Recent groundbreaking research associates repeated physical complaints, such as headaches, joint pains, and tummy pains, with anxiety, depression, and even disruptive behavior disorders in children. Helen Egger, M.D.'s study at Duke University looked at nearly 5,000 boys and girls ages nine to thirteen and assessed these physical complaints and psychiatric symptoms. Nearly two-thirds of the girls with an anxiety disorder had one or more of these physical complaints. More than two-thirds of the girls with stomachaches and headaches met the criteria for an anxiety disorder. Depressed girls were four times more likely to have headaches and nearly thirteen times more likely to have muscle and joint pains than girls who were not depressed. For boys, muscle and joint pain was associated with emotional disorders, and depressed boys were ten times more likely to have these pains than boys who were not depressed.

The take-home message from this important study is that boys and girls who have recurrent physical complaints may benefit from a comprehensive psychiatric evaluation. Specific physical complaints—muscle and joint pains at least three times a week in boys and girls and headaches that last for at least one hour and occur at least once a week in girls—may be useful cues to depression.

Action Plan

Construct a timeline of your child's physical complaints. Note the type of complaints and when they occurred, as well as how severe they are. On a separate line, write down anything significant that happened in the child's life at that time, from an illness in the child or the family to problems at school to troubling personal relationships. For example, you might note that your son's stomachaches started three days after his grandpa died, or the day before he brought home his report card, or the day after he had a fight with his best friend.

Fill out the Monthly Mood Chart (see page 7), paying particular attention to the physical symptoms section. Look for patterns or connections in your child's life that are related to physical and emotional symptoms. Notice any differences between weekends and weekdays, the various seasons, vacation time versus the school year, or the time of a teen's menstrual cycle. Also look at trips away from home, including sleepovers, and the absence of a parent. Sleep and appetite are also very important, so record how well your child has been sleeping and what he or she eats. For example, some children who eat lots of sugary foods before bedtime may be up all night. Others become moody after eating chocolate.

If you do notice connections, first discuss them with your spouse, then your child and, if applicable, with your child's teacher or pediatrician to develop a game plan to help your child.

Action Points

1. Connect the timing of your child's physical symptoms with what's going on in his or her life.
2. Pay particular attention to the time of day or week or season the symptoms appear.
3. Discuss the symptoms with your child and spouse, and if need be, get professional help to deal with them.

CHAPTER 3

How the Mind
Connects with the Body

*M*uch of how a child's body reacts depends on the brain. The latest research suggests that experience plays a huge role in how the brain develops and how genes for certain diseases are expressed. Just as changes in diet and exercise can help prevent you from getting heart disease if it runs in your family, good parenting is one of the "environmental factors" that can positively affect your child's behavior. It probably does this on a neurological basis. For example, if one identical twin has anxiety attacks (a neurological problem), the other twin (who inherited the same genes) will be much more likely than a nontwin to have anxiety attacks. This finding suggests that anxiety attacks are, in part, genetically based. However, more often than not, the second identical twin will not have anxiety attacks. The second twin's life experiences and environment may somehow modify this predisposition to anxiety attacks!

Children who go through the death of a parent or their parents' divorce may be more likely to have panic attacks. This experience of separation changes the way their brains develop. Chimpanzees in captivity show something similar. If mothers are intermittently separated from baby chimps to forage for food, the mothers appear anxious and their babies grow up to be unusually shy for their species.

On the other hand, many children identified at an early age as being shy or behaviorally inhibited turn out not to be shy at all. Why is that?

Some researchers think that life experience plays a key role. Parents can't control everything, but they do have some control. For example, they can send a child to preschool or arrange for play dates. You don't need to be a perfect parent. It's your pattern of behavior that can lead a child in the right direction, with the help of the principles presented in this book.

This chapter teaches you how to evaluate your children's physical complaints with examples of how I do this in my practice. I focus on the most common types of physical complaints: headaches, stomachaches, and joint pains. You will learn about the interface between the mind and the body, and how to ask your child the questions that provide the information you need to help identify and treat these problems.

You can learn how to think about, and not just react to, your child's behavior. I do this all the time with my patients in a more complicated way. If parents complain about their child's behavior, I help them understand why the child is doing what he or she is doing, which is what you do when you go to the doctor for medical complaints. If your child has stomach pains, you go to the doctor to find out whether it's a virus or an ulcer or some other problem. People are just not used to using this technique for nonmedical symptoms. The good thing is that you don't need a CAT scan to diagnose emotional symptoms.

Is It Serious?

Parents often ask how to know when a symptom is serious. Parents often disagree about whether something is abnormal or not. They may be unsure whether they should see a specialist. To many, psychology or psychiatry seems an inexact science. Anyway, your child's complaints seem to be the same as other kids', who seem to be okay.

Medicine may at times be more of an art than a science, and psychiatry is becoming less and less so. Ask yourself the following precise questions to find out what's bothering your child:

How intense is the symptom?
How frequently does it occur?
How long does it last, and how long has it been going on?
How much does it affect the child's functioning and thinking?
Can the child somehow alleviate the symptom and feel better?

Does the symptom seem to occur out of context, such as an
apparent stress headache that happens when the child is
not stressed?

When I talk to a child, I ask about home and family life, school, and
how things are going with friends and other activities. Whenever a child
has a physical complaint, it's important to know how he or she has been
feeling generally over the previous weeks and months.

Often, I'll find a pattern of stress-related physical symptoms. For
example, the child is better on the weekends and worse during the week,
or a child is always sick on Monday mornings.

I also look for patterns within the family. In some families, the main
mode of communication is complaining about symptoms. That's how
people get attention or communicate with one another. Who's suffering?
Who's in pain? A whole family may be oriented toward stress-related
symptoms, and the children may all have stomach pain and headaches.

Whenever I ask about pain, I use a scale that the child can relate to,
such as coding the pain on a scale of one to ten, with one being mild
and ten being the worst imaginable. With younger children, I use a
"visual" scale of a series of faces showing progressively more distress. I
ask the child to point to the face that best shows how he or she feels.
Other times, I use a drawing of a child's body and ask the child to color
in the areas that hurt, using red for the areas that hurt the most. I got
these techniques from psychologists who work behaviorally with children
in pain, notably Ken Gorfinkle, Ph.D., who works with me at Children's
Hospital of New York. With any pain complaint, it's important to know
whether pain-free periods occur, and whether sleep and rest make the
pain go away.

Headaches

When your child suffers headaches, ask what the headache feels like, such
as whether it's a throbbing, burning, stabbing, or a tight, squeezing pain,
and where in the head it hurts. This information is particularly important
since about one-third of children with migraine headaches have difficulty
describing the quality of their pain. Different types of headaches, from tension to cluster to migraines, cause different types of pain and in different

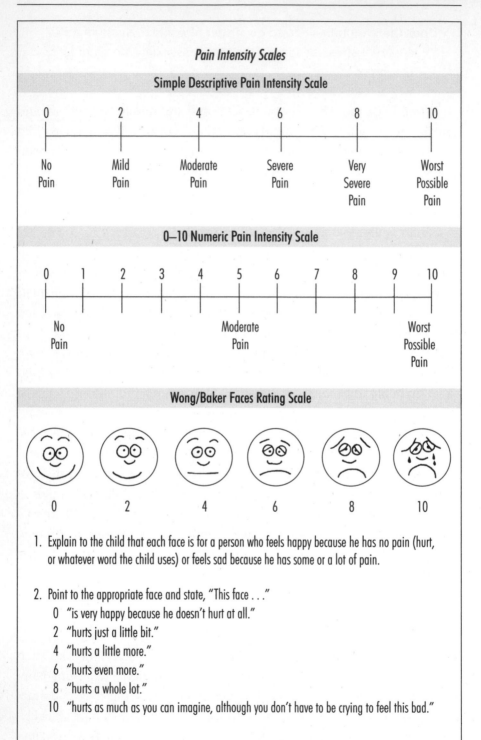

Pain Intensity Scales

Simple Descriptive Pain Intensity Scale

0	2	4	6	8	10
No Pain	Mild Pain	Moderate Pain	Severe Pain	Very Severe Pain	Worst Possible Pain

0–10 Numeric Pain Intensity Scale

0	1	2	3	4	5	6	7	8	9	10
No Pain					Moderate Pain					Worst Possible Pain

Wong/Baker Faces Rating Scale

0   2   4   6   8   10

1. Explain to the child that each face is for a person who feels happy because he has no pain (hurt, or whatever word the child uses) or feels sad because he has some or a lot of pain.

2. Point to the appropriate face and state, "This face . . ."
   0   "is very happy because he doesn't hurt at all."
   2   "hurts just a little bit."
   4   "hurts a little more."
   6   "hurts even more."
   8   "hurts a whole lot."
   10 "hurts as much as you can imagine, although you don't have to be crying to feel this bad."

places in the head. It's also important to know whether you can tell the child has a headache. Does the headache affect what the child is doing? Does it get worse when the child exerts himself or herself? If so, it might be an exertion headache. Does the child get sick to the stomach and/or vomit? Do lights or noise bother him or her? Is the child's vision affected? For example, ask, "Do you see differently? How?" Yes answers might suggest a migraine headache. Migraines tend to run in families, so it's important to find out if anyone else in the family has them. If headaches occur only on Mondays or before tests, they may be associated with stressful events, and need to be watched closely to make connections to stress.

Headache Checklist

- ❒ Does the headache feel like throbbing? burning? stabbing? or a tight, squeezing pain?
- ❒ Where in the head does it hurt?
- ❒ Can you tell when your child has a headache?
- ❒ Does the headache affect what the child is doing, or get worse when the child exerts himself or herself?
- ❒ Does the child get sick to his or her stomach and/or vomit?
- ❒ Do lights or noise bother him or her?
- ❒ Is the child's vision affected? If so, does he or she see differently?
- ❒ Does anyone else in the family have headaches?
- ❒ Is there a pattern to when the headache occurs?

Stomachaches

You can go through a similar process for stomachaches to help sort out stomachaches associated with syndromes such as irritable bowel from other more serious conditions. Keep in mind that parents must always have their pediatrician rule out a medical cause for particular symptoms. Looking at psychological or emotional contributions is something done *only* once symptoms have been medically evaluated.

Stomachaches often occur in conjunction with depression and anxiety. For example, children who jump up and down when they are in pain may not be suffering from disease in the GI tract, which will often make children remain quite still. Pain symptoms tend to be most concerning when they move away from the center of the abdomen and become more localized. The classic example is the lower right abdominal pain associated with appendicitis. It is important to follow the development of a pain symptom, though, since appendicitis, for example, often begins with pain in the center of the belly, and then moves down to the lower right side. Also note whether your child has recurrent stomachaches on the same day or at the same time each day. Try to associate the timing of the stomachache with what's happening in the child's life.

If you push on your child's stomach and it hurts when you release, the child may have a serious internal infection. This phenomenon, called rebound tenderness, happens when the peritoneum, which lines the gut, extends again after being pushed down, and needs to be checked out by a doctor. Changes in eating or bowel habits may also signify medical problems such as irritable bowel syndrome, Crohn's disease, or a malignancy. Bloody diarrhea or stool is always a significant concern, and should be evaluated immediately by a physician. A child who has battles over food or who retains stool, however, may have some other emotional problem, or at least one that could be helped by behavioral techniques that a pediatrician, psychiatrist, or psychologist can teach your child.

Different foods may also cause more pain because they affect the stomach differently. Some common foods such as nuts, eggs, and wheat may cause food allergies. Milk may upset the stomach of a child with lactose intolerance. And a child with ulcers may have problems eating spicy foods. Ulcer pain is typically felt fifteen to twenty minutes after eating due to the surge in acid production.

Stomachache Checklist

☐ Does the child jump up and down when he or she is in pain?
☐ If you push down on the child's stomach, does it hurt when you release your hands?
☐ Is the child eating and going to the bathroom normally?
☐ Does the child have a fever?
☐ Does the stomachache feel different at different times of the day, or on different days of the week?

❐ Do different types of food affect the stomachache differently?

❐ Is the stomachache worse on an empty stomach or a full stomach?

Joint Pains

Similarly, you can conduct an initial investigation to learn about the nature of your child's joint pains that are not associated with disease or injury of the bones or associated structures, which separates them from orthopedic problems. For example, if a joint or limb is swollen, red, warm, and has a visible cut near it, it's most likely infected. If your child can't move easily, or a limb is weak, numb, or sensitive to touch, he or she may have a serious nerve injury, which needs immediate medical attention. Similarly, if the joint pain is on both sides of body, it might be more than a simple ligament strain or muscle pull; it could represent more diffuse illness or rheumatological disease. Diffuse complaints such as these, in the absence of disease, may be related to stress.

Joint Pain Checklist

❐ Is the joint or limb swollen? Red? Warm? Have a visible cut near it?

❐ Is it difficult for the child to move?

❐ Is the limb weak, numb, or hypersensitive to touch?

❐ Is the pain on one side or both sides?

Emotional Behaviors, Physical Symptoms

Certain factors lead me to believe that emotional problems may be associated with physical symptoms. These include:

• Physical complaints seem to be way out of proportion to normal. The child's level of function or physical complaints change from one situation to the next; for example, depending on whether another family member is around.

• Fear clearly seems to interfere with the child's efforts to get better.

• Inconsistent functioning from day to day; for example, a child who one day can walk and the next day can't, even though the amount of pain hasn't changed.

- There is a "secondary gain," or some advantage that the child is not conscious of, to remaining ill. Typically, I see this in a child recovering from an illness who has missed a considerable amount of school. These children are either perfectionists who can't tolerate the anxiety of catching up or children with learning or social difficulties who feel extreme stress at school. Parents may unwittingly reinforce this behavior by paying more attention to the child's role of being sick.
- The child has a prior history of similar syndromes or other family members do. Interestingly, in some cases, a child mimics the true illness of another family member. One of my patients complained of acute pain in her foot while she was taking an exam the day after her mother fractured the same foot. Another child developed pseudoseizures (not true "electrical" seizures) after an uncle died from seizures.
- A child fails to recover despite what appears to be appropriate treatment.

Painful Complaints, Emotional Factors

Pain complaints may be affected strongly by emotional factors. When parents can't tell where painful symptoms are coming from, their children may suffer unnecessarily. They often miss out on social engagements, as well as going to school. Find out whether the pain began after a traumatic or stressful event or whether stress makes the symptoms worse. Loud pain complaints may seem to be out of proportion to what caused the pain. Or maybe your child seems to gain some benefit from the excessive pain. Such situations indicate that something is underneath the pain symptoms that you need to look at.

Pain Checklist

- ❏ Did the pain begin after a specific trauma or stress?
- ❏ Is a disability or handicap way out of proportion to the child's pain?
- ❏ Does the child have a clear secondary gain from the pain?
- ❏ Does the worsening of symptoms follow stressful events?

Action Plan

Once you have noted where your child's pain is, go through the appropriate checklists and try to identify the source of the pain with the information you have gathered.

Use the checklists to sort through your child's complaint and give you a sense of how much other factors may be influencing your child's pain. If nothing seems medically wrong according to your pediatrician, look for other conditions that often go along with headaches and stomachaches, such as depression or anxiety. Other things to look for include conduct problems, overactivity, and attention problems.

Any persistent complaints should be brought to your pediatrician's attention, who can work with you to find the right course of treatment. Treatment may include ways to relieve the pain symptoms through stress reduction, medications, and behavioral changes. If these solutions don't help alleviate the pain, and no medical problem appears to be the cause, then you may need to consult with a child psychiatrist for an evaluation. Take along your checklist information to help arrive at an appropriate game plan for treating your child's pain.

Action Points

1. Identify the source of your child's pain using appropriate checklists.
2. Get a sense of what factors may be influencing your child's pain.
3. Look for other conditions that may accompany headaches and stomachaches, such as depression, anxiety, conduct problems, overactivity, or attention problems.
4. If pain persists, see your pediatrician for treatment, which may include stress reduction, medications, and behavioral changes.
5. If necessary, consult with a child psychiatrist for an evaluation, and bring your checklist information along with you.

CHAPTER 4

Should I Send My Child
to School Today?

I got a call from Maxine because her daughter Patty, a socially awkward eleven-year-old who in some ways had compensated by focusing almost exclusively on her schoolwork, was complaining of abdominal pain, wasn't eating, and did not want to go to school. This situation had occurred repeatedly during times of stress. Maxine had taken Patty to the pediatrician many times, only to be told that there were no symptoms of any illness to be worried about.

Maxine asked me, "Should I have her exempted from a big test this week?" I thought that wasn't a good idea. Patty's symptoms seemed to be due to school stress. Staying home from school would only reinforce her pain symptom since it helped her avoid the stressful situation. Patty was an excellent student and had no learning disability. My recommendation was to have Patty complete all of her assignments, get some extra help studying for the test, and go to school. Avoiding school would just increase the stress associated with Patty's fear about keeping up, and make it harder for her to return. I encouraged her to go on school trips and to parties with friends. I met with her a few times and used a type of psychotherapy designed to focus on how social factors lead to mood problems. I also referred her for some group psychotherapy known as a "social skills" group, to help her overcome her nervousness around other kids her age. To help her reduce her abdominal pains and stress, I taught her a rhythmic breathing and imagery exercise. She successfully completed the school year with almost perfect attendance. Although she still complained of occasional stomachaches, Patty said she had "gotten used to them."

Translation: "Nobody likes me, which makes me nervous about being around other children. I worry about getting bad grades, and all of this just makes me depressed."

We used to think that children faked stomachaches and headaches to get out of school or to be manipulative. For years, this idea guided parents' responses. They might get angry and irritated and send their children to school with little empathy. While not a completely bad approach, it might ignore a subtle message about a child's emotional state, or even lead to the symptoms' getting worse. Or overanxious parents might focus too much on physical symptoms. They may let a child stay home from school, repeatedly, and miss the true message, which might have to do with stress over something at school or even depression. Then staying home from school becomes the reward.

This chapter debunks the myths surrounding complaints of aches and pains on school days. In the old days, doctors might have said a child had a nervous stomach, meaning that stress or something in his or her mind was creating the pain or perception of pain. Now we know there is likely something very different going on.

"I Don't Want to Go to School"

Going to school is usually an exciting time. But some children may react with fear or panic, and regularly feel sick from stress or complain of minor physical ailments and want to stay home from school. Most commonly, children don't want to go to school when they are faced with new challenges, for example, entering elementary or middle school. Leaving the safety of their parents and the sanctity of home may paralyze them with fear. The panic may come from leaving home rather than being in school, and often a child may become calm once he or she is in school.

Sometimes, a child will refuse to go to school after spending some time at home. A young child, in particular, may become closer to you during a summer vacation, school break, or brief illness, and become reluctant to return to school. Or stressful situations, such as the death of a pet or relative, a change in schools, or a move to a new neighborhood, may precipitate a similar reaction.

What are the typical symptoms of "school refusal"? Your child may complain of a headache, sore throat, or stomachache as he or she is getting ready for school, or just before it's time to leave for school. The symptoms may subside if you allow the child to stay home, but may reappear the following morning before school starts. Some children may simply refuse to leave the house or have severe tantrums when forced to go to school.

Refusing to go to school is common among children with separation anxiety disorder. These children may have an unreasonable fear of school for a variety of reasons. They may feel unsafe being apart from their parents, or worry excessively about their parents or about harm to themselves. They may be afraid of the dark. Some become clingy or shadow their parents around the house. Others may have difficulty going to sleep or have nightmares. Still others may have exaggerated fears of animals, monsters, or burglars.

Children who have persistent fears that they do not "grow out of," and that go untreated, are at increased risk for potential long-term effects, such as continued anxiety or panic disorder as adults. Children may also develop serious educational or social problems if they stay away from school and their friends for long periods. School refusal can be difficult for parents to cope with, but it can be treated successfully, if need be, with the help of a child psychiatrist or psychologist. Refusal to go to school in an older child or adolescent is generally more serious, and often requires more intensive treatment, which may include psychotherapy as well as medication.

Learning to Be Sick

This section sets forth a unifying theory about how children's bodies can become conditioned to feel pain or sickness. Children who are terribly stressed about a challenging situation may develop behaviors, such as vomiting, which begins with some biologically based sensitivity of their gastrointestinal tracts to the effects of stress. Even after the illness or whatever caused the pain is gone, the child may continue having the symptoms, not consciously, but because the child's body has been conditioned neurologically.

Eric Kandel, M.D., believes that any conditioned behavior is biologically mediated. Dr. Kandel won a Nobel Prize for discoveries crucial to the understanding of the normal signaling function of the brain and how disturbances in signaling can give rise to neurological and psychiatric diseases.

In his research, Dr. Kandel used the sea slug, a creature with relatively few, but very large, nerve cells, which allowed him to demonstrate the fundamental ways that nerve cell connections are altered. He trained the sea slug to produce two types of anxiety, one a conditioned fear, the other a chronic generalized anxiety. When he gave the animal repeated shocks to its tail, and a few minutes later a weak touch, it would overreact to the mild stimulus, much as people with chronic anxiety overreact to only mildly threatening situations. Dr. Kandel found that this chronic anxiety state has a completely different molecular basis, and requires the synthesis of new proteins within the animal's nerve cells. Certain genes are turned on or "expressed." That begins a cascade of activity ending in the production of a protein that promotes the growth of new connections between nerve cells, physically altering the wiring of the animal's primitive nervous system.

We now believe that a similar physical change occurs in human brains, not just when we are anxious but when we are learning and remembering. So when you help a child learn to deal with anxiety, molecular changes within the child's body probably occur. This concept puts a completely different spin on what changes in behavior mean and how they come about, and opens up new avenues of investigating physical symptoms. Modern molecular biologists will continue to study emotion and memory by zeroing in on specific genes, finding the ones, for example, that are active only in the amygdala, the part of the brain that is critical to fear and anxiety. Their goal is to determine which genes are critical to anxiety and then to develop drugs to reverse the effects of the proteins made following instructions from these genes.

The Sickness Seesaw

I like to imagine a sick child on a seesaw. On one side are forces that promote health and recovery; on the other, forces that perpetuate illness.

These forces may be biological, such as an infection or a medication; or they may relate to the environment, such as a child who tends to receive more attention when he or she has physical complaints. In some cases, the child receives more reinforcement for playing the "sick role" than for being well. For example, the mother of a sixteen-year-old girl who has chronic, unexplained abdominal pain has left her job and essentially become a twenty-four-hour nurse for her daughter, who is on "home instruction" and does not attend school. The two of them spend each day together, becoming more isolated from the rest of their lives, yet at the same time existing almost symbiotically. As the daughter spends more and more time away from the "normal" social circles of a high school junior, and more time out of school, it becomes much more stressful for her to return to "normalcy" than to remain at home with her mother. For her mother, who has given up her career to stay at home with her daughter, stepping outside this nurse role becomes quite challenging.

Assuming that your child is being treated correctly for an illness and is recovering, other things can affect your child's motivation for leaving the sick role behind. Until being well and getting better means as much, if not more, than being sick, the forces that maintain symptoms and disability may outweigh the forces of recovery. Many forces compete on each side, promoting either the sick role or the well role. Parents need to carefully review what's on each side so that they can help tip the balance toward wellness. Loading up the wellness side may mean, for example, that your child goes back to school three days after having the flu, if the doctor says the child is well enough to return, rather than being out for three weeks.

You can learn how to analyze a situation and to load up the wellness side of the seesaw. Take a good look at yourself and the way your family is functioning. Make sure your child gets enough rest, eats right, takes vitamins, and exercises. When dealing with any school situations—both social and academic—teach your child coping strategies for fears and anxieties.

Just Say No TV, No Computer

Jane called me at home in a panic one morning to say that her fifteen-year-old son Colin wouldn't go to school. Colin had been sick for a few days with a cold and had a history of refusing to go to school. He often complained of medically unexplained symptoms that would repeatedly disappear, including joint pains. I suggested that she tell him he could stay home only if he visited the pediatrician and had genuine signs of illness. And he couldn't watch TV or work on the computer. We also set up a 100 percent attendance requirement, barring a definite illness verified by the pediatrician. Colin decided to go to school that day and did not miss any days the rest of the semester. He began to participate in a group run by the school guidance counselor to talk about his feelings of self-consciousness.

Translation (subconscious): "The only way I can get out of being around other children is to be sick or hurt. Even though I have to miss school, it's worth it."

What do you do when your child won't go to school? First, parents must identify physical symptoms to make sure that they are not missing a medical condition. A savvy parent can usually tell when a child, particularly an older child, is truly ill. Visit your pediatrician to rule out a physical illness.

If you sense that the reward of staying home is greater than the reward of going to school for your child, point out that there's not going to be anything fun about staying home. Make it less appealing to be home, and insist that your child make up work missed from school. Then you need to delve deeper to find out the source of the problem and develop ways to modify the situation to relieve any stress. For stress reduction techniques, see Chapter 15.

"You Just Want to Get Back at Me"

Nine-year-old Ned had a habit of dawdling in the morning as he prepared for school. His parents had to constantly check that he had finished his breakfast, dressed himself, and brushed his teeth. His mother, Kathy, a high-powered attorney, always dropped him off at school on her way to work. "He just wants to make me late for work. It's his way of getting back at me because he's angry at me," she told me when she brought him in for a consultation.

I found Ned to be warm, friendly, and quite engaging, though a major power struggle had been set up between him and his somewhat controlling mother. He felt criticized and bad about himself for disappointing her. "The whole thing makes me mad at her and myself," he told me.

What's more, he was always anxious when he had not completed written assignments at school, putting them off until the last minute, and then struggling to do them. I checked with his third-grade teacher and it turned out that Ned was having problems, particularly with writing. The school psychologist uncovered difficulties with his visual-spatial and fine motor functioning, which clearly contributed to his problems with writing, organization, and paying attention. She suggested that he see a specialist.

Ned's parents became less angry when they saw that his difficulty getting things together in the morning was not a personal affront to them. Some tutoring helped Ned to organize his schoolwork. I recommended that he use a computer for his written assignments, and I helped the school accept this. His parents helped him organize his daily tasks into manageable chunks, with handy reminder lists. I suggested that they encourage and reward him for his efforts. Within several weeks, the mornings were running more smoothly in the household. Ned was much more on top of his schoolwork and even his writing showed improvement.

Translation: "I'm not just trying to make your life difficult! I'm doing the best I can, but I lose track of things. I'm having trouble getting my homework done because I can't write."

When a child doesn't want to go to school, try a different approach than simply reacting angrily. School attendance is mandatory if a child is not truly ill, but it is also important to find out the underlying reasons why a child might not want to go to school. Parents are prone to personalizing, taking an I-can't-believe-you're-doing-this-to-me attitude. In most instances, the child is not trying to "get" the parent. Underlying stresses may turn into family turmoil. Be a detective and try to uncover what's going on below the surface. Unreasonable fears about leaving home for school can be successfully diagnosed and treated. Don't hesitate to seek professional help, first from your pediatrician and, if necessary, the school psychologist or another mental health professional.

Action Plan

If your child refuses to go to school, the first question to ask is whether there is any possibility that your child gets something out of missing school. Is going to school more stressful than staying home? It turns out that many children with recurrent abdominal pain are

excellent students. Parents should understand that this is an unconscious process—the child isn't consciously faking symptoms. In fact,
it seems likely that there is something different in the GI tracts of
these kids, which makes them more prone to what specialists call
"visceral hyperalgesia," or heightened pain sensitivity of the organs in
the GI tract. Stress seems to influence these symptoms, and along
with genuine physical illness, such as a GI bug, can set off a cycle
of continued pain even after the initial illness is gone. A common
misconception among parents is that their child likes school and is a
good student, so there's no need to worry. But the child might still
be under extreme stress at school. So take those stomachaches seriously and investigate whether there is an emotional component.

Your child may be in conflict about attending school. On one
hand, the child wants to go to school, but on the other hand, doesn't.
The final decision about what your child does depends to some
degree on which side of the sickness seesaw is less stressful, and
how firmly you set limits. Unless the child is obviously sick, I strongly
suggest that you compel the child to go to school, though at the same
time it is important to continue medical follow-up and medical treatment of symptoms. For example, some children are helped by medicine to reduce spasms in the intestines or stomach acidity. Seek
medical treatment for symptoms that are uncomfortable to your child,
but don't keep your child out of school unless the pediatrician says to.
Especially when symptoms become chronic, as abdominal pain in
kids often can, it is important not to let your child begin to see himself or herself as disabled. This psychological transformation can be
devastating to the developing identity of your child. Even for a serious
chronic medical condition, you should emphasize adapting to and
coping with the illness, and being as normal as possible. Such children will attend school, social functions, and even play sports if possible. The approach to a chronic condition should be geared to
rehabilitation not convalescence. It is for this reason that doctors
often recommend physical therapy for children who have been sick
and home for a while, to help rebuild the decline in conditioning that
invariably accompanies being out of commission for a few weeks.
The process is similar to that of an athlete recovering from a muscle
sprain by slowly exercising the injured area, and tolerating the dis-

comfort associated with it. Avoidance is a common response to a stressful situation. Try to find out why your child is upset about school.

Hanging out with friends is a strong pull toward school. But a child who has been sick may be ambivalent about returning. The child has schoolwork to make up, and may be anticipating having to field uncomfortable questions about why he or she missed school. A child who had been doing well at school may be quite nervous about how well he or she is really doing in comparison to classmates. One way to help assuage this fear is to bring schoolwork home to allow a child to keep up as much as possible during the illness.

Once you flesh out what the conflict is about—another child is bothering your child on the school bus or there's a problem with a coach, teacher, or bully—then try to figure out how to address the issue. For a school bus problem, call the bus company, and speak to the appropriate teachers. If you have a bully problem, talk to the school principal. For more problem-solving technique involving bullies, see Chapter 9.

Going to school may be stressful not only for what goes on in school but also from the stress of leaving home. Your child may have separation anxiety. Ask yourself: Has a parent been sick? Is your child nervous about being away from home because he or she fears having an anxiety attack? Is your child afraid of getting sick in school? Essentially, does your child feel safer at home? More information on separation anxiety can be found in Chapter 6.

Children who have separation anxiety often have parents who have separation anxiety. Are you nervous when your child is away from you? Make sure you are not getting something from your child's being home. Do you feel safer when your child stays home from school? Remember, you are probably the largest influence in your child's life. If you suggest that your child stay home because of every little sniffle, the child will begin to believe that he or she really is too sick to go to school. Take a hard look at your own contribution. If you think that you may have separation anxiety, and if you don't mind involving the school, talk to the school psychologist about your own feelings. Or seek some psychological help from a private counselor.

The more attention you pay to illness behaviors—feeling sick, withdrawn, not participating, complaining about symptoms, and feeling disabled—the more your child can use them. On the other hand, if you reinforce wellness behaviors—returning to activities quickly, participating even when they don't feel 100 percent, and showing confidence in your child's vitality and ability to recover—can tip the sickness seesaw toward wellness. The more attention you pay to wellness behaviors, the better your child will function, even when sick. Take a positive attitude and offer encouraging, hopeful statements, such as, "You can do this," "You'll feel better soon," and "Stick with it." Believe in your child's ability to be well. A parent has to believe in a child's ability to function. On the other hand, if a parent either explicitly or implicitly does not believe their child can return to normal function, the child will pick up on this, and may not try as hard. Even in situations where a child has a bona fide medical illness, a parent's faith in a child's ability to nevertheless try to live as normally as possible can go a long way toward motivating a child to push himself or herself to the limit. Active coping statements and strategies, optimism, and an unrelenting belief in your child can help your child see things in a positive way.

Action Points

1. Take stomachaches seriously and look for the underlying emotions.
2. Try to find out why your child won't go to school, and address the issues.
3. Assess whether your child—or you—has separation anxiety.
4. Load up the wellness side of the Sickness Seesaw.

CHAPTER 5

Talking to Your Pediatrician—
How to Avoid Unnecessary Workups

took my two-year-old daughter Logan to the doctor a few months ago because she wouldn't walk. She said her hip hurt, but when little kids don't walk, there's always something wrong. Our pediatrician examined her, but couldn't locate the source of the pain. While at the doctor's office, Logan complained of ankle pain. The pediatrician said that sometimes ankle pain can be referred to the hip, and that's why Logan felt the pain there.

Over the next few days, I began to think, "What if the problem doesn't resolve? Maybe Logan needs a workup by a rheumatologist." I was tempted to call a pediatric rheumatologist colleague for a complete battery of tests. Instead, I spoke again to our pediatrician, who said it did not really look like juvenile rheumatoid arthritis, which was one of my fears. Sure enough, a week or so later, Logan was fine. We never did find out exactly what caused the problem, probably some minor injury from twisting her foot or stepping on something, but it went away by itself.

Translation: "I wish I could tell you why I can't walk, but I just can't; something hurts me."

When a child looks sick, parents want to know how to make things better. They usually call their pediatrician to find out what they can do to ease any discomfort and whether they need to take the child in. This chapter suggests what questions to ask the pediatrician, how to make judgments about symptoms and become a well-informed parent, when to rely on the doctor's opinion, what to do if you get conflicting opinions, and how to get a second opinion, when necessary. With guidance, parents can go through the medical system with a different perspective about how illnesses affect their children, and themselves, and use their child's doctor as a tool to get the most appropriate treatment.

Recognize How Symptoms Evolve

Lisa took her eight-year-old daughter Sara to the doctor because of complaints of headache pain. "We just moved here, and Sara was out of school for much of last year. We really thought it was largely due to stress," Lisa told the doctor, "and our old pediatrician reassured us the headaches probably weren't anything to worry about." Her new doctor asked Sara whether the headache pain was similar to what she had felt before, and she said that it wasn't, that it felt different from her usual I'm-stressed-out headache pain. For one thing, it was on only one side of her head. Sara was also sick to her stomach and sensitive to light when she had these headaches. Lisa chimed in, "Migraines run in my family." so the doctor ran some tests and determined that Sara was having migraine headaches. He prescribed one of the new medications for migraines, and referred her to a behavioral psychologist, who taught Lisa some relaxation techniques to ward off an impending attack, and went over her nighttime routine to help her get to sleep earlier.

Translation: "These headaches feel different. It's just hard for me to explain how."

Much of the art of a doctor's diagnosis comes from the patient's medical history. As a parent of a sick child, part of your job is to relate the child's medical history to the doctor, both the pertinent positives (such as pain) and the pertinent negatives (such as no blood in the stool). This information helps the doctor make a diagnosis, and helps the child get better care.

Typically, interactions between pediatricians and patients last only ten to fifteen minutes, with the pediatrician often talking more with the parent than the child. Parents quickly have to explain the child's symptoms, when they began, how long they have lasted, and other relevant information. In bringing these details to the doctor's attention, parents can guide the doctor's thinking process to find out what's going on.

A lot of what doctors and parents do is to recognize patterns. Instinctively, you follow the evolution of a symptom. Purely physical symptoms are obvious: your child started coughing on Sunday, and she's still coughing a week later. Parents can also learn how to investigate their child's potential emotional factors. When parents understand these factors, their children will have fewer medical tests and miss less school, and both the children and their parents worry less about something being seriously wrong.

When symptoms become prolonged, when they don't follow typical patterns of normal childhood illnesses, and the pediatrician has evaluated the problem sufficiently, one thing to consider is that the child may feel some secondary gain or advantage to being sick, as discussed in Chapter 4. The attuned parent may identify stresses that coincide with the onset of the symptoms.

Trust Your Doctor

When it comes to a sick child, parents must rely on their pediatrician's judgment. Doctors focus on objective signs and symptoms, and how the child functions at home and school. Symptoms such as a headache and feeling tired, but without a fever, could be due to a cold. If the symptoms don't seem to be getting better, then it's appropriate to ask for your pediatrician's opinion. A good pediatrician might say, "Well, this sounds a lot like the flu I've seen going around, and it may take a couple of weeks to clear."

If the symptoms continue to linger, then the doctor is obliged to do some baseline testing, for example, draw blood to look for mononucleosis or Lyme disease. A lot depends on the history and a physical exam—Does the child have joint pains? Does he have a belly ache?—and the pediatrician's judgment.

Because of an understandable anxiety about their child's health, many parents may want to see another doctor or a specialist. They may start worrying about other diagnoses after doing research of their own.

Using your pediatrician as the gatekeeper—the person in charge of coordinating your child's workup and for talking to other specialists, if necessary—prevents your child from being subject to too many workups from too many specialists.

The Dangers of Doctor-Shopping

Usually pediatricians treat general problems and refer you to specialists for more serious matters. A potential pitfall is when parents don't agree with their pediatrician and then get an opinion on the side, which their pediatrician never hears about. In this case, the pediatrician's impressions, as well as laboratory and test data, could be quite useful to the physician rendering another opinion.

In the worst-case scenario of doctor-shopping a child sees several specialists in the hospital and gets worked up multiple times because the doctors have not talked to each other. When one doctor coordinates all of the workups and evaluations, diagnosis time is shortened and that doctor can help parents decide when their child has had enough testing. Assessments of vague symptoms ("I just don't feel well.") or physical complaints ("My legs hurt.") that are not associated actual physical conditions are difficult.

Follow Your Instincts

On the other hand, parents must also follow their instincts, particularly if they disagree with their pediatrician. Most parents know when something is wrong with their child. They can just tell. If your gut instinct says there's more going on with your child, discuss this with your pediatrician. A good pediatrician will do his or her best to address your fears. Sometimes, this might involve additional tests or a second opinion. Don't be afraid to be proactive. Honest, open communication between you and your child's pediatrician is key.

Parents sometimes worry that the doctor will be insulted if they get a second opinion, though actually, when done collaboratively, a second opinion may be welcome.

Action Plan

If your child is sick, make a list of questions to take to your pediatrician about the patterns of the illness. You need to ensure that the doctor recognizes any patterns between the symptoms and stressful events in your child's life, recurrent symptoms that have been worked up before, or symptoms that don't follow typical patterns. The list might include: Could these symptoms be related to stress? Is there something wrong with my child? How will you find out? At what point do we consult a specialist? My child's in pain, what can I do to make him feel more comfortable? If my child is sick, are there psychological techniques that might help relieve her distress?

To help recognize patterns, keep a diary of your child's symptoms to take to the doctor and to get a clear sense of how the symptoms or illness may have evolved. Recording the symptoms will also help you avoid the risk of "overmedicalizing" a problem, that is, making more of it than it really is.

If you can, try to hold down your own anxiety about your child's being sick as you talk to the doctor. A visit to the doctor is nerve-racking enough as it is. It's important for parents to shield children from their anxiety because it can be infectious. A nervous child may worry that something "really bad" might be wrong or will happen to her, which may undermine the doctor's treatment. If you are anxious, it may be better to discuss your child's condition with the child out of the room to avoid making the child even more anxious. Parents should also be conscious of the impact on the child of expressing their concerns and worries about the illness. A parent's refusal to accept that psychological factors do exist may influence how the child reacts to your pediatrician's recommendations. Since psychological factors are very common in childhood illnesses, parents need not feel insulted if their child exhibits them. The presence of a psychological involvement in illness has nothing to do with the parenting skills. Everyone, young or old, has a psychological response to being sick. I am merely suggesting that parents tune into this, to help speed up your child's recovery, or at the very least, your child's adaptation to the physical problem.

Therefore, if you don't agree with the pediatrician's diagnosis or treatment recommendation, don't hide it. Discuss it openly with the pediatrician. If you agree to disagree about the diagnosis or treatment, ask for a referral for a second opinion. Let the pediatrician know you respect his or her opinion, but you want to gather more information. You might say something like, "I want someone else to give me an opinion of what might be wrong and how to treat it." If you do confer with other doctors, have them report to your pediatrician to keep him or her in the child's treatment loop.

If you have concerns and reservations, be proactive about your child's care. If your child is diagnosed with a condition or given a medication, do some research through medical resources easily found on the Internet or in bookstores. Go to the list of medical foundation Web sites in Resources at the end of this book to see whether any are appropriate for your child's condition or suggested treatment.

Action Points

1. If your child is sick, bring in a list of questions to ask your doctor and a diary of the symptoms to help recognize the pattern of the illness.
2. Try not to be too anxious at the doctor's office to help dampen your child's anxiety.
3. Be willing to accept a psychological influence in your child's illness.
4. If you don't agree with your doctor's diagnosis, make sure to discuss it openly.
5. Do research about your child's condition on the Web or through books.

PART II

Finding Out

What's Going On

CHAPTER 6

What's in the Body
May Be in the Mind

Molly seemed to be a happy fourteen-year-old. Sometimes she was more irritable than most girls, but her mother Joan chalked that up to Molly's innate judgmental temperament. While Molly enjoyed after-school activities, when she entered seventh grade she lost enthusiasm for school. She let her schoolwork slip a little and thought of her classmates as "spoiled." "Molly's the smart one in her clique, and the one the others come to for advice," says Joan. "We thought her behavior and mood were attributed to temperamental teenage angst. We didn't associate migraines, stomachaches, fatigue, or sleep problems to depression."

Molly scared herself by drinking too much at an unchaperoned party. The next day, she told her mother that, according to a test in a teen magazine, she thought she might be depressed, and she wanted to see a counselor. After six sessions, her psychiatrist couldn't find any significant source for Molly's melancholy, though they began to work on the distortions in thinking and social isolation that were part of her depression. Her psychiatrist suggested that she might benefit from a medication evaluation, which brought her to me. After a thorough evaluation, I agreed that she might recover more quickly with the addition of an antidepressant. "Since taking the medication, Molly has been less irritable and more cheerful," says Joan. "We all notice more smiles and less uptight behavior."

Translation: "My physical symptoms were just my body's way of telling me I was depressed."

This chapter goes through a head-to-toe review of all the emotional or psychiatric problems that manifest themselves physically. The key is to look at the child as a whole person. Parents need to take a broad view of what is happening to their children. This doesn't mean ignoring individual symptoms. Parents can become members of the medical specialist's team by providing impressions that lead to the proper diagnosis. And early recognition of these problems in most cases leads to early treatment that prevents further problems later in life.

Mental Illness

A recent study of hospital admissions for children and teens at the University of Washington shows that while overall hospital admissions decreased in the 1990s, mental illness became the leading cause of hospitalization for this group. Pediatric consultant Michelle Garrison's analysis of admission records at the university hospital showed that total hospital admissions were down 34 percent for school-aged children five to fourteen years old and adolescents ages fifteen to nineteen years. But in her presentation at the 2002 Pediatric Academic Societies meeting, she reported that hospitalization rates for mental illness had increased by 20 percent in school-aged children and remained steady for teens. During the study period, mental illness accounted for 12 percent of the hospital admissions for school-aged children and 20 percent of the admissions for teens. One-third of their time spent in the hospital was attributed to mental illness.

This very important study raises some questions: Is this a national trend, and if so, what is causing this trend? Is this a reflection of us as parents, of our society, or of the stresses on our children? Do we have enough resources to help parents and pediatricians recognize mental health problems and intervene early, when necessary? I hope that this book will help parents recognize problems early on and have them evaluated before they reach the kind of crisis proportions that require hospitalization. Also, we need to look as parents, and as a society, at what might be leading to emotional problems in our children, and act to prevent them.

Depression and Anxiety

The two most common psychiatric illnesses seen among both adults and children are depression and anxiety. When children are identified early, parents can do something that makes a difference and prevent the development of more serious emotional problems later on. Unfortunately, pediatricians identify less than one-third of children with emotional problems, and less than half of those identified get referred to mental health specialists

Accidents, a major cause of death in children and adolescents—from falls, fires, drowning, and car accidents—are more likely when a child and/or family has emotional problems. Children with chronic illnesses are twice as likely to have emotional difficulties.

A diagnostic quiz can help parents identify when a child may be depressed or anxious, or both. For example, Monica, a fourteen-year-old girl, dropped down to 76 pounds after losing more than 30 pounds because she was vomiting so much. She had a feeding tube put into her stomach to get some calories into her, even though she had no clear disease in her gastrointestinal tract. She was finally diagnosed with severe depression and anxiety. Following psychotherapy and treatment with medication, she gained 35 pounds in three months, and was well two years later.

When thinking about the severity of symptoms, parents need to consider the number of symptoms, frequency, duration, and number of places they happen; the child's functioning with friends, in school, during activities, and the impact on the family; the child's burden or suffering, including the intensity of suffering, its duration, and any limitations of activities; the danger to the child or others; and how much the symptoms intrude into the child's development or daily activities.

A proper evaluation by a trained mental health professional should include an extensive history provided by the parents, information provided by the school and/or contact with the child's teacher(s), an appropriate medical evaluation, interview with the child, and certain clinical questionnaires that can help assess symptoms of mood disorders.

More Than "the Blues"

All children get a brief case of "the blues," but true depression is different. Severe depression is a serious medical illness that must be treated.

Depressed children feel irritable or have a depressed mood for two weeks or more, and may also have the following symptoms, according to the American Academy of Child and Adolescent Psychiatry (AACAP):

- Change of appetite with either significant weight loss (when not dieting) or weight gain
- Change in sleeping patterns (such as trouble falling asleep, waking up in the middle of the night, early morning awakening, or sleeping too much)
- Loss of interest in enjoyable activities
- Loss of energy, fatigue, or feeling slowed down or burned-out
- Feelings of guilt and self-blame for things that are not the child's fault
- Inability to concentrate and indecisiveness
- Feelings of hopelessness and helplessness
- Recurring thoughts of death and suicide, wishing to die, or attempting suicide

Children with depression may also feel irritable, grumpy, and bored, and may have vague, nonspecific physical complaints, such as stomachaches, headaches, or muscle or joint pains. They may be absent from school frequently; talk about running away from home; shout out suddenly, complain bitterly, start crying, or become irritable for some unexplained reason; show lack of interest in playing with friends, or become socially isolated; express a fear of dying; become extremely sensitive to rejection or failure; or exhibit reckless behavior.

The diagnosis and treatment of depression in children can be a major challenge. Many children and teens suffer from depression, a disorder that can have far-reaching effects on their functioning and adjustment. Depressed children may have personal and social difficulties that persist long after an episode of depression. Depressed teens also have an increased risk for substance abuse and suicidal behavior. Unfortunately, depression often goes undiagnosed because the signs of depression may seem like the normal mood swings of growing up. In addition, doctors are often reluctant to prematurely "label" a child with a diagnosis of depression. Yet, early diagnosis and treatment are important, if not essential, since the large majority of depressed children can be helped.

In addition, depressed children may find it difficult to identify or describe their feelings or moods. For example, children typically don't complain about how bad they feel, and may instead act moody and cranky. Parents may interpret the child's actions as misbehavior or disobedience. In fact, research shows that parents are even less likely to identify depression among teens than are teens themselves.

Far more scientific studies of depression among adults have been conducted than among children. A handful of large-scale studies, most of them conducted in the last four to five years, have evaluated the safety and effectiveness of antidepressant medication for depression and anxiety in children. We need larger trials to determine which treatments work best for which children and more studies to show how to incorporate these treatments into routine care. That's why it's important to involve a child psychiatrist or psychologist in the evaluation, diagnosis, and treatment of a child who is suspected of having depression.

Scope of the Problem

About 5 percent of children and adolescents suffer from depression at any given point in time, according to the Child Academy. Research also shows depression is occurring earlier in life, and it often persists, recurs, and continues into adulthood. Children who become depressed may also have more severe depression as adults. Young depressives often have other disorders, such as anxiety disorders, along with illnesses such as diabetes.

The increased risk of suicide among depressed children may rise, particularly among adolescent boys, if the depression is accompanied by conduct disorder and alcohol or other substance abuse. Suicide is the third leading cause of death among young people ages fifteen to twenty-four, following unintentional injuries and homicide, according to the National Institute of Mental Health. It is very important for doctors and parents to take all threats of suicide seriously. Early diagnosis, which includes an accurate evaluation of the child's suicidal thinking, and limiting access to lethal weapons such as guns and medications may be the best suicide prevention of all.

Screening Tools

If a parent suspects a child is depressed, a further evaluation should be done. This may include interviews with the child, parents, teachers, and anyone else who may have pertinent information about the child's moods. Parents can help identify major sources of stress for their child and help develop better coping strategies. During treatment, several tools are available to doctors to track depressive symptoms in children, including the Children's Depression Inventory (CDI) for ages seven to twelve and, for teens, as well as the Beck Depression Inventory, and the Adolescent Depression Rating Scale (ADRS).

Risk Factors

Both boys and girls appear to have about the same risk for developing depression. Teenage girls, however, may be more at risk than teenage boys. Depressed children are more likely to have a family history of depression and often have a parent who became depressed at an early age. Other risk factors include: teenage cigarette smoking; stress; the loss of a parent or loved one; attention, conduct, or learning disorders; chronic illnesses, such as diabetes; abuse or neglect; and other trauma, including natural disasters.

Treatment

Depression treatment for children often combines short-term psychotherapy, medication, and targeted interventions at home or in school. In general, treatment is continued for at least six months after all depressive symptoms stop to prevent a recurrence.

Certain types of short-term psychotherapy, particularly cognitive-behavioral therapy (CBT) and interpersonal psychotherapy (IPT), can help relieve depression in children and adolescents. CBT helps children refocus their distorted views of themselves, the world, and the future. Studies show that two-thirds of depressed teens may go into remission with CBT and faster than with either supportive therapy or family therapy. Other related forms of focused, problem-solving psychotherapy such as IPT target interpersonal features of depression, and also appear to be effective. Psychotherapy may also help a child who has been pre-scribed antidepressants to take them, and a child may be able to partici-pate more in therapy if physical symptoms, such as low energy, sleep problems, and loss of appetite, are improved with medication.

For adults, clinical studies clearly show a combination of antidepres-sants and psychotherapy is an effective treatment for depression. How-ever, using medication to treat children is more controversial. Many doctors have been understandably reluctant to treat depressed children with psychotropic medications because there has been little evidence, until recently, about their effects on children.

However, researchers have conduct randomized, placebo-controlled studies on children over the past few years. Two of the newer antide-pressant medications that are selective serotonin reuptake inhibitors (SSRIs) have been shown to be safe and effective for the short-term treat-ment of severe and persistent depression among children. So far, con-trolled studies have shown good results for the SSRIs fluoxetine and paroxetine. Large-scale studies are still needed for SSRIs. Tricyclic antide-pressants should generally not be prescribed for children or adolescents with depression *because they have not been shown to be effective in younger patients*. The American Academy of Child and Adolescent Psy-chiatry recommends that medication can be an effective part of the treat-ment for childhood depression, especially when it is combined with psychotherapy in a comprehensive treatment plan.

Other Types of Depression

Although less common in young children, bipolar disorder (also known as manic-depression) can appear in both children and teenagers. Bipolar dis-order involves unusual shifts in mood, energy, and functioning. A child may exhibit either manic or depressive symptoms at first, then switch to the other. The depressive symptoms in a bipolar child or adolescent are similar to those of depression in a patient who has no history of mania. The manic symptoms may include unusual happiness or silliness or extreme irritability; an overly inflated self-esteem; a great increase in energy; going for days with little or no sleep without tiring; talking too much or too fast; changing topics too quickly; not being able to be inter-rupted; attention moves constantly from one thing to the next; or a disregard of risk. Children with bipolar disorder are more likely to have parents with the disorder, which suggests a genetic component to the disease.

Young children with bipolar disorder often experience rapid mood swings and cycle from depression to mania several times within a day, so called "rapid cycling." Children with mania are more likely to be irritable and prone to destructive tantrums, rather than being elated or euphoric. Bipolar disorder accounts for a large proportion of children's psychiatric hospitalizations. Some 20 percent of adolescents with major depression develop bipolar disorder within five years of the onset of depression, making it tricky to treat an initial episode of depression, since antidepressant treatment in a child who is a "latent" bipolar may "switch" the patient into mania.

Teens with bipolar disorder display a combination of extremely manic and depressive moods. Their highs may alternate with their lows, or, for some, their moods may change so quickly that they both appear at almost the same time.

Other psychiatric disorders may exist alongside the bipolar illness, making a thorough evaluation essential. An irritable, aggressive teen may be depressed, have a conduct disorder, may be abusing drugs, or have attention deficit hyperactivity disorder (ADHD). Any child who appears to have serious mood symptoms and exhibits severe ADHD-like symptoms should be evaluated to rule out a co-existing mood problem, such as bipolar disorder, particularly if there is a family history of mood disorders. This evaluation is particularly necessary since the stimulants often prescribed for ADHD may worsen manic symptoms.

Bipolar Disorder: A Warning about Antidepressants

Using antidepressants to treat a child with depression who has bipolar disorder may induce manic symptoms. While it can be hard to determine which young patients will become manic, the likelihood is greater among children who have a family history of bipolar disorder. Parents should be aware of the signs and symptoms of mania so that they can recognize them immediately. Several factors in a depressed teen seem to make it more likely that he or she may turn out to be manic, including family history of mania, previously getting manic on antidepressants, having psychotic symptoms, severe psychomotor retardation (being slowed down), and having a rapid onset of depressive symptoms.

Dysthymia

Children can also have dysthymia, a lower level of depressive symptoms that last for at least one year. This less severe, yet typically more chronic, form of depression is accompanied by at least two of the symptoms of major depression. Dysthymia often precedes a major depressive disorder, but treatment may prevent the child's condition from deteriorating to more severe illness. Children with dysthymia are at high risk of developing a more serious depressive illness later on.

When to Worry about Worrying

Children also get anxious about lots of things. A recent Dutch study led by Peter Muris, Ph.D., from Maastricht University found that almost 70 percent of children aged eight to thirteen years reported that they worried now and then. These worries were generally about school performance, dying, health, and social contacts, and they occurred an average of two to three days per week. The worries often interfered with tasks and were hard to control. And worry, anxiety, and depression were found to be strongly related. The information in this section should help parents tell the difference between an everyday worry and an anxiety disorder.

Intense, unpleasant feelings or physical symptoms when anticipating danger or problems probably mean the child has an anxiety disorder. The Child Academy describes five types of anxiety disorders found in the *Diagnostic and Statistical Manual of Mental Disorders, Fourth Edition.*

> **Separation anxiety disorder:** Excessive anxiety concerning separation from home or loved ones. The youngster may worry excessively, be reluctant or refuse to go to school, or afraid to be alone or to sleep alone. Repeated nightmares and complaints of physical symptoms (such as headaches, stomachaches, nausea, or vomiting) may occur.
>
> **Generalized anxiety disorder:** Excessive anxiety and worry about events or activities, such as school. The child has difficulty controlling these worries and may also be restless, tired, tense, and irritable, and have difficulty concentrating and sleeping.
>
> **Panic disorder:** Unexpected, recurrent panic attacks. These sudden, intense feelings of apprehension, fear, or terror are often

associated with feelings of impending doom. They may be accompanied by shortness of breath, palpitations, chest pain or discomfort, choking or smothering sensations, and fear of "going crazy" or losing control.

Phobias: Persistent, irrational fears of a specific object, activity, or situation (such as flying, heights, animals, getting a shot, seeing blood). They can cause the child to avoid the object, activity, or situation.

Selective mutism: Failure to speak (though the child actually can) in social situations usually involving nonfamily members, such as teachers or other children. Selective mutism is probably a prototype for social phobia in adults.

Anxious children are often overly tense or uptight, and their worries may interfere with daily activities. They may need a lot of reassurance. Children with anxiety are often quiet, compliant, and eager to please, which makes it difficult to diagnose. Parents should be alert to the signs of severe anxiety so they can intervene early to prevent complications. It is important not to discount a child's fears.

If you are concerned that your child may have an anxiety disorder, consult a child psychiatrist or other qualified mental health professional. Severe anxiety problems can be treated, and early treatment may help prevent the child from losing friends, failing to reach his or her potential, and feeling low self-esteem. Treatments may include a combination of individual psychotherapy, family therapy, medications, behavioral treatments, and consultation with the school.

It's a Family Affair

Parents also have to be suspicious if they have had depression or anxiety. The children of depressed parents are more likely to be depressed, too. Adults with anxiety disorders usually had them as children, though most children with anxiety disorders grow up to be okay; most childhood anxiety is transient.

There is a strong relationship between anxiety disorders in parents and anxiety and depression in their children. Many children of parents who have panic attacks have higher rates of separation anxiety. Also, some children with depressed parents have separation anxiety. While the specific disorder isn't transmitted genetically, the underlying risk is.

"I'm Not Sad or Anxious"

While the diagnostic criteria for depression and anxiety are great, children who are depressed or anxious often aren't aware of it, or won't admit it. Parents sometimes have to go with how their children behave and how other adults and their friends see their children. For example, a child may complain of unexplained physical symptoms and won't attend school, do his schoolwork, or see his friends, but denies feeling sad. His parents might suspect he's depressed based on his withdrawal from social activities, inability to function or to enjoy things, concentration problems, and loss of energy.

A child who has stomachaches and constantly leaves class to visit the nurse could be anxious about school, though she denies feeling worried. Her parents might have to investigate her academic and social functioning to help figure out where she feels stress. If she has no medical disorder, the stress has to be coming from somewhere.

Other Psychiatric Disorders

A handful of other psychiatric disorders may also cause physical symptoms, which are portrayed through the following anecdotes.

Tourette's syndrome—Mike, a seven-year-old boy, has been clearing his throat and sniffling for almost one year, and has been treated with a variety of allergy medicines. His pediatrician conducts a thorough review of his history and failure to respond to allergy medicine; it becomes clear that he is having frequent tics. He is eventually diagnosed with Tourette's syndrome.

Pseudoseizures—Lance, a fifteen-year-old boy, has frequent spells in school where he loses consciousness and has an increase in his blood pressure. He doesn't respond to smelling salts or rubbing hard on his breastbone. He is admitted to an epilepsy monitoring unit, where it is shown that his brain waves are normal during these episodes, and he is diagnosed with pseudoseizures. He is found to have depression, a learning disability, and tremendous anxiety about school. Following psychotherapy, treatment with anti-depressants, and a change in his school program, his spells stop.

Pain syndrome—Nancy, a twelve-year-old girl, had been seen by multiple medical specialists, including neurologists, orthopedists, and rheumatologists, for her severe, unremitting joint pain. She required constant opiate medication over two years. Her pain was found to be due to a pain syndrome that was associated with a serious depression. With treatment, including physical therapy, psychotherapy, antidepressants, and hypnosis, she improved radically and was gradually taken off pain medication.

Body dysmorphic disorder—Chai, a sixteen-year-old boy, is preoccupied with one of his eyes being slightly wider than the other. His parents have taken him to several eye doctors and plastic surgeons, requesting that his "defect" be repaired. Chai has covered all of the mirrors in his home and refuses to leave the house due to his self-consciousness. The doctors find that one eye is, indeed, open several millimeters wider than the other, but that this is physiologically normal, as no one's face is perfectly symmetrical. His diagnosis is called body dysmorphic disorder, which may be related to obsessive-compulsive disorder. But Chai and his mother refuse psychiatric treatment, continuing to look for a surgeon who will treat him.

All of these disorders require a complex approach that combines medical, psychiatric, or behavioral interventions that may involve medication. Often physical therapy, and sometimes family therapy, is also an important adjunct. I believe that these so-called psychiatric disorders undoubtedly have neurological roots. Body dysmorphic disorder, for example, is probably related to obsessive-compulsive disorder, which appears to be a neurological-based problem involving nerve cells in a region of the brain called the basal ganglia, and which responds to the same antidepressant medications used for OCD.

Medication Questions

Before a child receives medications, which are commonly prescribed for children with the types of disorders described in this chapter, parents should ask the doctor to answer such questions as: For what emotional problems is the medication appropriate? How can psychiatric medicine be used in medically ill children and adolescents? What are the common medications and dosages used, and how long do they take to work? What are the side effects to watch out for? How do you know if the medicine is helping? How long should a child be on psychiatric medication? What are the important drug interactions to watch out for?

The Next Generation of Drugs

New drugs that affect the stress hormone cortisol may be the next generation of medications for depression and anxiety. Depressed patients tend to have elevated levels of cortisol. New findings hint that drugs that inhibit cortisol release may represent a novel class of both antidepressants and antianxiety drugs. These drugs, known as corticotropin-releasing factor antagonists, probably act on deep structures of the brain. Psychotherapy is also known to reduce anxiety and depression, probably by acting on the brain area where thinking occurs. The combination of drug therapy and psychotherapy works better than either one alone, probably because of the impact on two important brain areas.

Environmental Programming

I'd like to present a provocative interpretation of how the brain responds to environmental programming. Parents can program their child's brain development by regulating exposure to stress, and promoting coping skills and activities that relieve stress. Severe stressors early in life, such as neglect or abuse, have been associated with anxiety disorders in adulthood. Researchers think that stressors may alter the brain circuits involved in the release of cortisol. Interestingly, successful treatment seems to normalize these brain circuits.

This evolving area of research has tremendous implications for all newborns, not just for abused children or those neglected by their mothers. It underscores the importance of recognizing and treating anxiety and depression. Parents who recognize stress in their children, and can help their children release the stress, may reduce their risks of anxiety and depression.

Action Plan

Familiarize yourself with the symptoms of depression and anxiety. Be aware that children who are depressed or anxious may not admit, or even be consciously aware, that they are being affected by their moods. For more information about depression and anxiety, go to the Child Academy Web site and Resources section of this book.

If you think your child is depressed or anxious, ask your pediatrician for an opinion, and, if necessary, get a referral to a mental health specialist. Take a list of your concerns along with you to the doctor's office. Make sure to note the signs and symptoms of mood changes, when they began, how much distress your child is in, how much this affects your child's functioning, whether anyone else in your family has ever had similar symptoms, and whether your child has felt this way before. Keep a symptom diary for one month, if you can, rating by the day your child's or adolescent's anxiety, irritability, and depressed or elevated mood on a scale of 0 to 3 (0 = normal, 1 = slightly abnormal, 2 = moderately abnormal, 3 = severely abnormal). Note any events that might have affected your child's mood.

In addition to not talking about being anxious, sometimes a child will go to all lengths to avoid anxiety-producing situations, and so will not be anxious. Think about symptoms that may be masked by your child avoiding a situation. For example, a child with separation anxiety who always sleeps with her parents at night may not exhibit separation anxiety at home, but may be very afraid to have a play date, be alone, or go to a friend's house.

Undiagnosed depression is a significant risk for a child's health and well-being. Don't be fooled into thinking that adolescents are not depressed. Many depressed teenagers grow up to become depressed adults, with a high rate of suicide and suicide attempts. With treatments now available, early identification is imperative to try to head off the consequence of depression among adolescents.

Many psychiatric disorders, for example, Tourette's syndrome, have patient treatment groups, Web sites full of good information, and Internet bulletin boards ready to share information with others. Try to find parents with children whose diagnosis is similar to your child's.

Ask your doctor, parent groups, or search the Web, or consult the list in the back of this book.

Take care to screen health care professionals, including psychiatrists, neurologists, psychiatrists, or pain specialists, who may treat your child. Be wary of a health care professional who sees a symptom as all physical or all psychological. Many of these complicated disorders have biological components and psychological factors that contribute to the severity of your child's symptoms. That's one reason why every reputable pain center has a consulting psychiatrist, who should be included in your child's care. Find out the practitioner's approach before committing to treatment. Ask about the kind of practice the doctor runs. Is it mainly psychotherapy or does the doctor just prescribe medicine? Does the doctor often see medically ill children? Even biologically based disorders have psychological factors; for example, tics are made worse when a child is anxious.

The best doctors are generally those who are identified by their colleagues. It's important to know where the doctor got his or her training. Sometimes patients request my professional resume, and I'm glad to send it to them. Ask about Board certification. For example, a child psychiatrist may be a member of the American Board of Psychiatry and Neurology. You'll find that doctors who work at major medical centers are more likely to be board certified. '

Familiarize yourself with how medications are used and the risks of medications through Web sites, your pharmacist, and a review of the drug's literature. One of the best books for parents about psychiatric medicine is *Straight Talk about Psychiatric Medications for Kids* by Dr. Timothy Wilens. This book provides up-to-date information that will enable you to understand fully what your doctor is recommending and what your options are. Be aware that psychiatric medications often have important interactions with other prescription drugs, as well as over-the-counter medications. Ask your pediatrician or pharmacist about drug interactions whenever a drug is prescribed. Make sure to mention all of the medications your child is taking, including homeopathic and herbal remedies, which may interact with prescribed medications. See Chapter 18 for more about the potential dangers of alternative remedies used in combination with prescription drugs.

The essential first step is to see a good diagnostician who will approach your child's symptoms with a broad view and help you formulate a treatment plan. Regardless of your child's illness, the plan should involve a team approach. In most cases, this approach involves more than just medicine. It might include psychotherapy, physical therapy, behavioral changes, and dietary changes. Parents should be an integral part of the diagnosis and treatment process.

Action Points

1. Know the signs and symptoms of depression and anxiety.
2. Get help from your pediatrician and specialists if you think your child is depressed or anxious.
3. Don't be fooled if your child says he or she is not depressed or anxious.
4. Use all resources available to you—your doctor, specialists, patient groups, the Web—to gather information about specific disorders.
5. Become familiar with the medications prescribed for your child.
6. Become a part of your child's diagnostic and treatment team.

CHAPTER 7

What's in the Mind
May Be in the Body

While many emotional disturbances have physical signs and symptoms that resemble a medical illness, the opposite is also true. Researchers have recently discovered "psychiatric" diseases that appear to be rooted in the body.

This chapter helps parents recognize when emotional symptoms may represent a true medical problem. A series of anecdotes helps guide parents from mistaking psychological problems for physical ones. Lyme disease can cause psychiatric manifestations, such as moodiness, attention problems, and depression. Strep infections can cause abrupt and severe obsessive-compulsive behavior, as well as tics. Hormone disorders sometimes mimic depression. Irritable bowel syndrome can lead to strong stress-related reactions. Chronic pain syndromes may be associated with depression.

Lyme Disease in Disguise

Paul, a fourteen-year-old boy from upstate New York, began to feel tired, develop concentration problems, and feel joint pains over the summer months. His parents and his doctor suspected that Paul had depression. While he didn't recall being bitten by a tick or developing a rash, Paul's blood tested positive for Lyme disease, and a spinal tap showed the disease had affected his nervous system. After treatment with intravenous antibiotics, Paul recovered fully.

Lyme disease has been called "The Great Imitator." Caused by a tiny organism that infects the brain and joints, this disease can cause psychiatric manifestations, such as moodiness, attention problems, and depression. But less than one-third of those infected with Lyme disease remember being bitten by a tick and do not develop the characteristic bull's-eye rash. Lyme disease has become a major public health hazard. However, few physicians are aware of how it may masquerade as a psychiatric illness. Lyme disease has few physical symptoms and doctors disagree over what constitutes a definitive diagnostic test. For example, different physicians may interpret the results of a common Lyme test (called the Western Blot) in different ways. One physician may say that the test is conclusive for Lyme, and another may say that it is not.

One problem with Lyme disease is that it is difficult to know exactly when a child was bitten by a Lyme-carrying tick and when the symptoms began. Because the flu-like symptoms may be mild and not very specific, the child or his parents may not realize the child has been bitten. So the child may have been infected for weeks before symptoms develop and antibiotic treatment begins.

If untreated, Lyme disease can affect multiple systems in the body and may cause neurological and psychiatric symptoms. In fact, Lyme disease has been associated with the new onset of obsessive-compulsive disorder (OCD). Some children who have Lyme disease that has gotten into their central nervous system (CNS) become moody, depressed, talk in negative terms, and worry that they won't get better.

After six-year-old Gabe was diagnosed with Lyme disease in his CNS, his parents brought him in to see me because he was having difficulty in kindergarten. "I feel stupid," said Gabe. I suggested to his parents that we look at Gabe's academic functioning and mood symptoms for a while to see if they were related to the Lyme disease or to his reaction to being ill. We also met with a neurologist because his mother thought Gabe had developed a tic. I consulted with Brian Fallon, M.D., a national expert in the psychiatric manifestations of Lyme disease. He noted that the kind of mood problems Gabe was having—feeling more depressed in the evening, for example—were not typical of Lyme disease. I suggested we treat him with psychotherapy and discontinue antibiotics, as I continued to reassure his parents that Gabe's moodiness was probably not due to the Lyme infection.

I also taught Gabe some strategies to use if he began feeling depressed. Using his imagination, he created a Super Gabe character and a Mr. Sad, an electrified embodiment of feeling sad. If Mr. Sad came back, Gabe decided he would shoot a cannon at him, douse him with water since he's electric, and imagine that he put electrical tape on all the wires in the house so that Mr. Sad could not get in from the outside. After a few months of treatment, Gabe was not feeling particularly depressed, and we gradually tapered off his therapy.

Lyme disease may also cause an autoimmune reaction—a reaction where the body fights itself—that leads to neurological and psychiatric symptoms. (See below.) My colleagues and I have identified two cases of children with OCD and/or tic disorders after they had been infected with Lyme disease and/or had a strep infection who could be classified as having this autoimmune reaction. Perhaps, as may be the case with strep infections, Lyme infection may cause the formation of antibodies that fight the infection, but mistakenly attack tissue in an area of the brain called the basal ganglia, resulting in symptoms including tics, and obsessive-compulsive behavior.

Strep Infections

Following a strep throat, Tierney, an eight-year-old girl, suddenly became obsessed with the thought that her hands were contaminated with germs, and she began to wash them compulsively all day long until they turned raw. She was diagnosed with pediatric autoimmune neuropsychiatric disorders associated with streptococcus (PANDAS). After receiving intravenous immunoglobulins, along with penicillin, her obsessions and compulsions went away.

The *Streptococcus* bacterium, which causes the strep throat epidemics seen especially in winter, can also cause abrupt and severe obsessive-compulsive behavior, as well as tics. Often, these behavioral changes and anxieties can be attributed to emotional factors or underlying psychiatric illness. Understanding the medical reasons for what looks like an obvious psychiatric problem is essential since treatment with antibodies, antibiotics, or blood-cleansing plasmaphoresis may be indicated, and the correct diagnosis is needed for proper treatment.

Brain Inflammation or Extreme Shyness?

Sam, a four-year-old boy, appeared to have stopped talking because he was shy, had a lisp, and was very competitive with his twin sister, Ryan. His history, however, was not really consistent with the selective mutism disorder, in which extremely shy children will not speak in public. His symptoms had followed an infection, which was accompanied by behavioral changes including increased sleepiness, moodiness, and strange behaviors such as licking things, and pulling on his ears. Though a renowned physician suggested the possibility that the child had become autistic, further studies including an MRI, EEG, and spinal tap, helped us postulate that the boy had a postviral encephalitis, or inflammation in the brain. After treatment with intravenous immunoglobulins, Sam began to talk again.

Selective mutism is a psychiatric disorder most commonly found in children. These children understand spoken language and have the ability to speak—they speak to their parents and selected people with whom they feel comfortable—but may not speak to others at home or in school, or at social gatherings. Many researchers think this disorder is related to severe anxiety and social phobia, but the true cause is still unknown. The majority of children who have selective mutism have parents or other family members who have extreme shyness, social phobia, or anxiety disorders, which suggests a genetic influence or vulnerability.

Most children with selective mutism want to speak, but anxiety, fear, shyness, and embarrassment make them unable to express themselves. The same behavior management programs used to treat phobias work well for selective mutism.

Hormone Disorders

Jamie, a sad ten-year-old boy, complained of severe obsessive-compulsive symptoms, including washing his hands and other rituals that took hours each day. He also had fatigue, memory problems, and had gained weight. I diagnosed him with obsessive-compulsive disorder (OCD). Interestingly, laboratory tests that I order for any child I place on medication showed that Jamie was not producing enough thyroid hormone. In addition to the OCD, he needed to be treated for hypothyroidism. His mood improved following treatment of both his OCD and thyroid condition. I later diagnosed hypothyroidism in his depressed sister the same way. It turned out to be a family condition.

Certain hormone disorders can mimic psychiatric illness. Both hypothyroidsim (low thyroid levels) and hyperthyroidism (oversecretion of thyroid hormone) can affect mood, and even cause psychotic symptoms, such as hallucinations. Thyroid dysfunction can also reduce the effectiveness of antidepressants. Hypothyroidism symptoms include sluggishness, mental dullness, feeling cold, or muscle cramps. Too much thyroid hormone may lead to symptoms of insomnia, nervousness, palpitations, and tremor. Many hypothyroid patients (predominantly women) have significant depressive symptoms, which are often accompanied by a significant slowing of movement and a mild effect on thinking. The association between depression and clinical hypothyroidism is generally well accepted. A higher-than-expected incidence of depression also occurs among patients with subtle, milder forms of hypothyroidism. Disorders of two other glands, the adrenal and the parathyroid, may also look like depression, and can also be picked up with routine laboratory tests.

Irritable Bowel Syndrome

Eleven-year-old Alex was a high-powered scholar-athlete who swam competitively. When I met her, she had been complaining of severe stomach pain and nausea for months and had missed a lot of school. Over that time, she had dozens of tests and seen a handful of specialists. Knowing that depression can also cause physical complaints that prolong recovery, her last specialist suggested that I consult with Alex.

We talked about all of the tests she had, and what was going on in her life. I discovered that her superior abilities had led her parents, coach, and herself to have extremely high expectations of her. Although she wasn't conscious of it, the stress to achieve was taking its toll. Amazingly, no one said she showed any signs of stress. Alex received pain management and stress-reduction techniques, physical therapy to help her regain strength, and a diet with increased bulk and more water. When her symptoms did not respond after a month and were continuing to completely disrupt her life, I prescribed an antidepressant. An intriguing treatment is one of the newer antidepressants that affect the hormone serotonin—selective serotonin reuptake inhibitors, or SSRIs. These medications may decrease spasms in the gut. The dose is usually one-half to one-third of that used to treat depression. Results can appear as quickly as in several days, or may take as much as ten weeks to be seen. Child psychiatrists are reporting success using SSRIs in kids with recurrent abdominal pain. In this case, Alex's stomach pain and nausea resolved several weeks later, and she returned to school.

Children with irritable bowel syndrome (IBS) truly have "different" intestines, which seem more likely to spasm in response to stress. Stressful events, such as the break up of a close relationship, often precede IBS. I have seen bouts of IBS among college students during final exams and young kids who were rejected by their peers. Poor coping styles, such as making everything into a catastrophe, and chronic stress can keep IBS going and going.

About half of adult IBS patients have a psychiatric disorder, which often precedes the development of the disease, so the patient's psychological state is key. In children with gastrointestinal pain, the symptoms often become chronic. Some 12 percent of all patients seen by primary care doctors turn out to have IBS. And the problem tends to run in families: two-thirds of these kids' parents and half of their siblings also have had abdominal pain.

The Pain of Pain

Juliana, a seventeen-year-old high school junior, had had knee surgery five years ago following a sports injury. She developed pain in multiple joints and complained of balance problems, dizziness, and headaches. As a result, her schoolwork suffered. Consultations with neurologists, rheumatologists, and orthopedists at three leading medical centers found no evidence that her symptoms were consistent with any known medical disorder, though one doctor did suggest it might be fibromyalgia.

When Juliana saw me, she was on a steroid to treat inflammation and narcotic painkillers. She admitted to multiple worries, and appeared quite depressed. I treated her depression with medication and psychotherapy, along with physical therapy, biofeedback, and hypnosis. Her steroids and narcotics were gradually reduced as her pain subsided. Six months later, she was without pain and attending school, with a bright mood.

The approach to treating a chronic disorder without an identifiable cure, per se, is to try to rehabilitate the person, to get them back to life, so to speak. This can be difficult, since kids often have troubling symptoms, such as pain. However, an empowering approach motivates and teaches the child how to control the symptoms, rather than letting the symptoms control him or her. This wellness model helps children avoid taking on the sick role—the psychological identity that children adopt when they start to see themselves as helpless, or worse, disabled. Regardless of the child's physical problem, the focus must always be on strengthening the body and the spirit. So much of what I see with kids with chronic physical symptoms are the secondary effects of being sedentary, such as deconditioning or muscle atrophy and weakness. We must make these kids strong and help them believe in themselves and their ability to overcome symptoms.

Action Plan

First, don't rule out a psychiatric problem because you think your child is faking it. In the twenty-first century, the underlying neurologic causes of almost all psychiatric disorders are under investigation. In fact, some of the leading experts for these problems are in the field of psychiatry. One leading expert on Lyme disease is New York–area psychiatrist Brian Fallon, M.D., who has also done extensive research about hypochondria, suggesting that it may be related to obsessive-compulsive disorder, which is probably caused by abnormalities in an area of the brain called the basal ganglia. Hypochondria may simply represent another type of obsession, and may respond to the same type of antidepressants as OCD (SSRIs). You shouldn't automatically shy away from a psychiatrist because of the potential stigma of having your child labeled as "seeing a psychiatrist." As I've shown in this chapter, specialists have the expertise to investigate serious mental health problems and, at times, come up with amazingly simple answers.

If you do see a child psychiatrist, find one with experience in dealing with physical symptoms. Not every child psychiatrist deals with medically ill children. Ask your pediatrician for a referral to one who does. Or contact your local hospital and find out which child psychiatrist consults with medically ill children.

Make sure to bring up your child's physical symptoms with the child psychiatrist during your first consultation. It's important to avoid getting into an either/or situation. A child's illness cannot always be attributed to either a psychiatric or a medical cause. A child may have some changes in cognitive abilities, and symptoms of moodiness—possible signs of Lyme disease—and not have Lyme disease. Such a child might become distressed over being ill and because of neurological changes, which hurt school performance and confidence, and make the child more nervous. So don't ignore the psychiatric for the medical. Get a thorough workup to ensure your child receives the best possible diagnosis and treatment.

Sometimes, you have to be an advocate for your child, but don't succumb to the pitfall of doctor shopping, that is, going to one doctor after another. Children with multiple, mysterious symptoms often are seen by more than one specialist. If you find yourself in that situation, don't talk about only one subset of your child's symptoms to each doctor. Give a comprehensive view of all of the symptoms to all of the doctors. It is crucial that all of the doctors involved in your child's care talk to each other and exchange information.

Pain clinics, found at many major medical centers, take such a multidisciplinary approach to treatment. A child psychiatrist may prescribe and coordinate treatment among a pain specialist and other people involved in your child's care, which may include a behavioral psychologist as well as a physical therapist. Rehabilitation, not convalescence, is the focus of therapy. These clinics generally offer integrated services that include pain medications as well as nonpharmacologic treatments such as behavioral intervention, including hypnosis. Your child may also receive a psychiatric medicine that works well for other problems, for example, an antidepressant for abdominal pain. As trusted colleague Dr. Boris Rubinstein notes, "the medicines don't know that they are antidepressants."

A twelve-year-old girl referred to me by the pain service with chronic joint pain and compulsive joint cracking (especially her knuckles) had a mother who was convinced this young lady had a "stealth virus" that was causing inflammation in her joints. These symptoms caused her to seek over thirty opinions from various specialists at different medical centers. She had kept the girl out of school for almost three years. After an extensive evaluation, it was determined that she did not have any neurological, infectious, or rheumatological disease. The child neurologist and I felt she might have a tic disorder, but that what was driving her symptoms was her mother's irrational belief that she was ill, which defied all medical explanation and evidence. When this situation was dealt with, the girl began to renounce some of these "inherited" beliefs. With psychotherapy and rehabilitation, she will hopefully be able to return full time to school.

If your child develops symptoms of depression or pain, use imagery—have your child imagine what he or she can do to feel better; distraction—play a game or read a book; or positive self-talk. These techniques will likely ease the symptoms and help your child feel better. Behavioral psychologists and developmental pediatricians are experts in using techniques such as hypnosis to ease pain in children.

Again, you can educate yourself about your child's diagnosis or treatment through the Internet and other sources located at the end of this book. I can't emphasize enough that your child needs integrated, multidisciplinary care. A child psychiatrist and other specialists, such as a neurologist, can work closely with your pediatrician to coordinate your child's collaborative care.

Each of these so-called emotional disorders requires a keen eye to see how they differentiate from true psychiatric problems. Parents must work first with their child's pediatrician to get an initial diagnosis, and then with specialists to uncover the true underlying cause.

Action Points

1. Be open to seeing a mental health professional for your child's condition.
2. Find a psychiatrist who deals with medically ill children.

3. At the first visit to a psychiatrist, describe your child's physical symptoms.
4. If you see more than one doctor, make sure that they all have all of the medical information about your child to coordinate care.
5. Look for a pain specialist at a major medical center.
6. For pain or depression, use imagery, distraction, and positive self-talk to help ease symptoms.

CHAPTER 8

How Your Child
Thinks and Speaks

att is an eleven-year-old whose sixth-grade teacher is constantly frustrated with his not listening and seemingly forgetting his assignments and books. His strict teacher tells his parents that she has decided to "teach Matt to be more responsible" by giving him all Fs. "Matt is bright when it comes to reading and math, but he obviously is capable of being more organized, and his handwriting is abominable simply because he is not careful," she says. Matt became quite demoralized, and after many angry discussions and fights with his parents about becoming more organized, he was even less motivated to do his schoolwork. "I am trying hard. It's just that no one appreciates that," he told me when he came for a consultation.

My first suggestion was to get psychological testing to determine Matt's strengths and weaknesses. While his verbal IQ was "superior," his non-verbal IQ, which measures things like the ability to write and to organize material presented both spatially and visually, was only "average." The greater than fifteen-point difference between Matt's verbal and nonverbal IQ suggested that Matt had a nonverbal learning disability, and that his difficulties organizing material and projects were neurologically based. Once Matt's teacher knew the nature of his problem, she began handing out written instructions for his assignments. He got help in his organizational and planning skills and with his note taking. He also learned to type, which helped him tremendously in completing his assignments.

Translation: "I'm not lazy, and I do care about my grades, but it's hard to pay attention and keep track of everything, especially in middle school when stuff is so much harder. Why is it that some things come so easy to me, and other things don't?"

Nearly 4 million school-aged children have learning disabilities, and about 3 million of them receive special education services, or about 5 percent of all children in public schools, according to the National Institute of Mental Health (NIMH). This number doesn't include the thousands of children in private and religious schools who have learning disabilities but receive few or no services, or those who don't meet the criteria established by public schools to receive special education services.

To help you understand how your child's thinking and speaking may affect school performance and social interactions, you can do an overall mini-assessment. This chapter includes a checklist so that parents can get a rough idea of their child's development. While the checklist helps you break development down into different domains, such as language, social skills, and physical abilities, you need to look at all of the areas as a whole. A child can be far ahead in one area, reading, for example, but actually have a significant problem with another, such as writing or athletics. This dichotomy can sometimes mislead even the most astute parent or teacher. This is because if a child seems bright in some areas, the assumption may be that he or she should be able to do well in all areas. In school, skills such as reading, writing, and math are generally emphasized. If a child has difficulty with "nonverbal" skills such as planning, organization, or visual-spatial skills, this may not be readily apparent because it is not "tested," per se, though it can cause a bright child to "not perform" well in a specific area, even if he or she is bright in that area. I like to think of these problems in computer terms. A child may have problems inputting data (vision, hearing, attention), in storage (memory), in central processing (problems processing material that is seen or heard, organizational problems, or other neurologically based problems that affect how your child processes information), and in output (problems with oral or written expression).

If your child has developmental problems, speak to your child's teacher, or get your child independently assessed by a psychologist who does specific testing. You can request that the school psychologist do this type of testing, or have it done privately.

Developmental Challenges Checklist

Does your child have:

❐ Problems learning how to read
❐ Problems learning how to write
❐ Problems learning how to count or do math
❐ Problems with organization
❐ Problems copying pictures or shapes
❐ Problems understanding or recalling things he or she sees
❐ Problems understanding or recalling things he or she hears
❐ No sense of cause and effect
❐ Problems with nonverbal cues
❐ Problems processing or understanding social cues or nuances
❐ Problems with physical boundaries or clumsiness
❐ Sensitivity to light, touch, or sound
❐ Repetitive or stereotyped behaviors
❐ Lack of empathy
❐ Difficulty with transitions
❐ Difficulty regulating mood
❐ Poor gravitational sense—that is, do they ever "tilt" to one side and/or have difficulty keeping balance

Learning Disabilities

Learning disabilities are neurological disorders that interfere with a child's ability to receive, store, process, or produce information. These disorders can affect a child's ability to read, write, speak, or do math, and can also interfere with social skills. Sometimes overlooked as "hidden handicaps," learning disabilities may go unrecognized or are often not considered serious until they are detected. Children with learning disabilities usually have normal intelligence. They try hard to follow instructions, concentrate, and be good at home and in school. But, despite their best efforts, they may not master basic academic skills and tend to fall behind their classmates. Some children with learning disabilities are also hyperactive and are unable to sit still, are easily distracted, and have a short attention span; this is not because of their learning disability necessarily, as they may also have attention deficit hyperactivity disorder (ADHD), which is NOT a learning disability. Others misbehave in school because they would rather be seen as "bad" than "stupid."

The impact of a learning disability can be relatively mild to severe. Learning disabilities often run in families. Their cause is believed to be subtle disturbances in brain structure and function that affect receiving, processing, or communicating information. For some, disturbances may begin before birth with errors in fetal brain development. Other factors that affect brain development include genetic factors; tobacco, alcohol, and drug use; problems during pregnancy or delivery; and toxins in the child's environment. While they are not cured per se, a child can learn to compensate for a disability and overcome areas of weakness.

The tragedy of undetected learning disabilities is a "snowballing" effect. For example, a child who does not learn addition in elementary school has little chance of "getting" algebra in high school. The more the child tries to learn, the more frustrated he becomes, and he may develop emotional problems such as low self-esteem due to repeated failure.

Learning disabilities can be divided into three broad categories, according to the DSM-IV: developmental speech and language disorders; academic skill disorders; and other disorders of motor skills or specific developmental disorders not otherwise specified. An NIMH booklet, *Learning Disabilities* (NIH Publication N. 95-3611, printed 1993; reprinted 1995), describes these disorders in detail, and is an excellent resource for getting help and sustaining hope.

Any child suspected of having a learning disability should have a comprehensive psychological and educational evaluation. By "psychological" evaluation, I am referring to aptitude tests that measure IQ, reading, and writing ability, for example. Educational evaluations generally measure achievement by giving specific tests. These evaluations are meant to help identify areas of relative strength and difficulty, and to help determine whether your child is eligible for specialized assistance in school. Evaluations can be arranged through the public school system at no cost, or through private clinics, private evaluators, hospital clinics, or university clinics. Some school districts may not automatically accept test results from outside sources. Check with your school district before getting an evaluation from a private facility.

If you have any questions about whether your child's thinking and speaking are age-appropriate, talk to your pediatrician. Your pediatrician can help you decide whether further evaluation is needed. Doctors can run screening tests to see whether a problem exists, such as a vision examination by an eye doctor, a psychological examination by a psychologist or psychiatrist, a hearing examination by an ear-nose-throat doctor and audiologist, or a language assessment by a speech and language specialist.

The treatment recommendation may include individual or family psychotherapy. Beyond overcoming any disabilities, the goal of treatment is to strengthen your child's self-confidence, and also help you and other family members better understand and cope with the realities of living with a child with learning disabilities.

Attention Disorders

Attention deficit hyperactivity disorder (ADHD) may occur along with learning disabilities. While estimates vary, approximately 3 to 5 percent of school-age children may have a type of attention disorder that includes such features as marked overactivity, distractibility, and/or impulsiveness, according to NIMH. These behaviors can, in turn, interfere with a child's ability to benefit from school, and often accompany academic skills disorders.

Some children with ADHD appear to daydream and are easily distracted. If they are quiet, their attention disorder may go unnoticed. They may be sent from one grade to the next without getting the help they need.

An attention disorder may be accompanied by hyperactivity, which happens more often in boys than girls. These children can't seem to sit still, act impulsively, run into traffic, or topple over chairs. They may blurt out answers in the classroom and interrupt their school lessons. In the playground, they can't wait to take their turn. They often get into trouble with their parents, teachers, and friends. This type of attention disorder is hard to miss, though it could be mistaken for "normal boy" behavior. The difference is that in ADHD, the hyperactivity is developmentally inappropriate, or not appropriate to the context, and impairs the child's functioning.

Even though a child is misbehaving or being difficult, it may be hard to know exactly what is wrong. At times, all children lose their attention, are easily distracted, act impulsively, or seem to be hyperactive. But ADHD children tend to display these symptoms and behaviors more frequently and severely than their peers, and in a manner *not* appropriate for their age. ADHD must begin before age seven, and tends to run in families, with about 25 percent of biological parents also having ADHD.

A child presenting with ADHD symptoms must have a comprehensive evaluation, particularly since other psychiatric disorders, including oppositional defiant disorder, conduct disorder, anxiety, depressive, or bipolar disorder, may accompany ADHD; in fact, seeing ADHD without another diagnosis is less common than seeing it along with other problems. Without the proper diagnosis and treatment, an ADHD child may fall behind in schoolwork, experience more failure than success, lose friends, and suffer criticism from teachers and family who do not recognize the problem.

Without the proper diagnosis and treatment, an ADHD child may fall behind in schoolwork, experience more failure than success, lose friends, and suffer criticism from teachers and family who do not recognize the problem.

Many ADHD children find that stimulant medications help them. Medications such as methylphenidate (Ritalin, Concerta, Metadate), dextroamphetamine (Dexedrine), or Adderall can improve their attention, increase compliance, and decrease hyperactivity and impulsivity. Other medications such as guanfacine, clonidine, and some antidepressants may also help. For more about the effectiveness of medications, see Chapter 16.

A combination of medical treatment and other approaches, such as cognitive-behavioral therapy, may provide the most effective treatment, according to the Multimodal Treatment of ADHD study, which is discussed in detail in Chapter 16. Cognitive therapy can help build up a child's self-esteem, reduce negative thoughts, and improve problem-solving skills, as well as help to control aggression and modulate social behavior.

Other methods that may help include social skills training, parent education, and modifications to the child's education program. Parents and teachers can learn management skills, for example, to issue instructions one at a time rather than making multiple requests all at once. Modifying educational goals can help address ADHD symptoms along with any coexisting learning disabilities.

ADHD should not be thought of as a disability, meaning that the goal should be adapting and compensating for whatever attentional and social challenges that exist. Your child should not hide behind his symptoms and must take responsibility for his or her actions, and the need to develop the skills necessary to be successful; he or she will rise to the level where you set the bar. If your child shows symptoms and behaviors that suggest ADHD, ask your pediatrician for a consultation and, if necessary, a referral to a child psychiatrist who can be more skilled in diagnosing and treating ADHD.

Asperger's Syndrome

According to the American Academy of Child and Adolescent Psychiatry, Asperger's syndrome is a pervasive developmental disorder that is characterized by problems in social skills and repetitive behaviors. Previously, Asperger's syndrome was often confused with autism or other developmental disorders. Asperger's children generally function at a higher level than autistic children, and must be carefully evaluated.

Many children with Asperger's syndrome have normal intelligence, and begin using words at age two, although their speech patterns may be odd. They often have a large split between their verbal and nonverbal IQ, with the nonverbal IQ being disproportionately lower. Most Asperger's children are loners and have difficulty playing with children. Some exhibit eccentric behaviors and a restricted range of interests, for example, being quite preoccupied with weather, maps, or counting. Children with Asperger's syndrome commonly have coordination problems and often need special education.

No one knows what exactly causes Asperger's syndrome, but there appears to be a genetic connection. Children with Asperger's syndrome are also at risk for other psychiatric problems including depression, ADHD, schizophrenia, and obsessive-compulsive disorder. Effective treatment usually involves a combination of psychotherapy, special education, behavior modification, family support, and possibly medication. The prognosis for Asperger's syndrome is generally promising. Many children with Asperger's syndrome finish high school, and while they may continue to have social problems, they often develop long-term relationships with family and friends.

Autism

According to the Child Academy, autism is a more severe developmental disorder, characterized by repetitive routines, odd, peculiar behaviors, communication problems, and a lack of social awareness. In most cases, an autistic child is identified by age three by the "classic" signs of with-drawal, aloofness, and failure to respond to others, or, in some cases, to even make eye contact. Autistic children may also engage in odd or ritu-alistic behaviors, including rocking, hand waving, or an obsession with maintaining order. Many don't speak, or if they do, speak in rhyme, echo others' words, refer to themselves in the third person as "he" or "she," or use peculiar language.

Autism can vary in severity from mild to severe. Some bright children do well in school, but may have problems adjusting socially. Others func-tion at a much lower level; mental retardation is commonly associated with autism. Occasionally, an autistic child displays an extraordinary talent in art, music, or math.

Like Asperger's syndrome, the cause of autism remains unknown. Current theories suggest a central nervous system problem.

An autistic child needs a comprehensive evaluation and specialized behavioral and educational programs, and may also benefit from medica-tion. Medication may target symptoms including compulsive behavior, rigidity, or attentional problems, for example, thought it does not treat the disorder, per se. Without a current cure, appropriate evaluation and treat-ment are important to help a child's development and reduce disruptive behaviors and symptoms.

Action Plan

Just because a child has done well in lower grades doesn't mean that a learning disability won't become apparent in upper grades when the work gets harder. That doesn't mean that your child is "stupid." Your child may be far advanced in one academic area, and not in another—a student who gets straight *A*'s in everything except English. It may seem as if your child is not putting in enough effort. But that may not be the cause of the problem. The work may be too hard to handle, and your child may shut down mentally because he or she is frustrated.

If there's any question about the way your child is learning, talk to your child's teacher. The teacher may recommend that you consult a learning specialist for a psychoeducational evaluation, which evalu-ates both aptitude and achievement. You can use this evaluation to help guide you, if something is identified. Along with a doctor's evaluation, you can come to a recommendation on treatment. For example, a child with organizational problems can use techniques to become more organized, including the use of color-coded folders, a date book, and written homework assignments that the teacher makes sure the child takes home. In some instances, a second set of books can be obtained and left at home. Some children may need tutoring or help from the school's resource room. If the school doesn't have the facilities, seek out a private tutor or therapy center.

Don't be fooled by a child's effort and motivation. I have often heard children referred to as "lazy." There is no such term in any textbook to describe the reason why a child is having problems, and this label is not only derogatory, but not useful in terms of finding ways to help. If "laziness" explained your child's problem, what exactly would be the treatment? Lack of effort can be caused by many things, including frustration, attentional difficulties, depression, learning disabilities, or dynamic issues in the family. Your child's functioning may be related to how well the child performs in a particular subject, as well as prior experience. For example, if your child has done poorly in math all semester, the following semester she may not put in the required effort. Try to find out what's going on beneath the effort problem. See things constructively and positively. If need be, seek help.

For potential developmental challenges, identify which domains are affecting your child's functioning. If you suspect a delay, then you may need a formal assessment by a pediatrician, mental health professional, or neurologist. Occupational therapy or physical therapy might also be part of the plan.

For cognitive functioning—reading, writing, math, organization, shapes, and memory—compare your child with others you know, or remember how an older sibling functioned at the same age. Ask your child's teacher how your child compares to his or her classmates. Most schools have formal teacher reports or teacher conferences that offer you an opportunity to discuss these matters.

Fine motor functioning involves such skills as tying shoes, buttoning, picking up and holding things, and manipulating small objects. You may see your child has problems getting dressed or holding crayons, paint brushes, or pencils. Again, your child's teacher should have great input into any problems in functioning.

Gross motor functioning—how your child balances, throws, catches, kicks, and is generally coordinated—is seen primarily through athletic activities. Watch how your child performs on a team or at an active party, for example, at a play space or on the playground. Check with teachers how well your child does in gym class.

Social functioning—how your child relates to peers, both at home and in school—can be identified by your child's relationships with others. Look at the child's interest in playing with other children, and the quality of the play. Does your child share and take turns well? Does the child simply play alongside other children without inter-acting, called "parallel play"? How about following rules, staying focused on the game, and tolerating losing? Some answers follow the child's developmental level. School-age children should be able to tol-erate losing a game and to follow the rules; preschoolers may not be react as well to losing a game. Preschoolers should be able to share in activities such as dress-up, playing with dolls or action figures, or games in the pool during the summer or sleigh riding in the winter.

Teachers are invaluable resources about a child's social func-tioning. Ask whether your child shares thoughts and interests with other classmates. Find out how well the child plays and interacts with others in the classroom.

Some children might have fine or gross motor functioning prob-lems, but no social problems. If you see delays in any area, or com-binations of areas, it's worth it to get more information. Talk to your pediatrician first. If the two of you identify something suspicious, then a consultation with a specialist may be in order. But first look beyond developmental disorders for signs of other problems. If functioning problems are associated with mood symptoms, it might be depres-sion. If your child is adjusting to a new situation, it could be stress from outside the home. On the other hand, if your preschooler has lost the ability to relate socially and seems "out of it," it could be an "autistic regression," but a neurological problem, such as seizures, for example, needs to be ruled out. If a relatively acute change in bal-ance, vision, thinking, speaking, or coordination happens with no rea-sonable explanation, or your child has frequent headaches or fevers, a neurological evaluation may be in order. In general, symptoms in two or more of the developmental domains warrants a neurological evaluation of the child.

Some children also have problems with sensory integration. They have a strange sensitivity to light, touch, or sound, or prefer to sit in certain postures or to lean against something or have something lean against them. Others have tactile sensitivities and prefer certain texture foods or types of clothing. While these preferences may seem to be based on compulsions—wearing the same red shirt every day—they may be sensory based. In this case, get an occupational therapy evaluation.

Various types of specialists can be very helpful for children with developmental challenges. Impairments in social functioning should be assessed by a psychologist or psychiatrist. Some children who have never developed socially may have the inability to pick up on nonverbal cues and nuances, or to make eye contact. A consultation with a neurologist may be in order since neurological illnesses such as metabolic or seizure disorders can cause these types of delays.

Gross motor problems generally require a physical therapy evaluation, and speech problems an evaluation by a speech therapist. Reading, writing, and math problems usually require psychological testing.

You can also look for nontherapeutic activities to help your child. For a gross motor problem, try karate or gymnastics. For a fine motor problem, art classes may be helpful. For social problems, teams or club activities, such as the Boy Scouts or Girl Scouts, can be helpful.

I want to stress that each child develops at a different rate. Don't be discouraged because your child is delayed in one or more areas. If you intervene early, your child may catch up. Early intervention also helps head off self-esteem problems since many children with developmental delays feel that they can't do as much as others. Always think about how your child may be thinking in all of these areas, and try to encourage him or her.

Another important consideration is how you will explain these types of evaluations and interventions to a child. I think it is important to always try to frame everything in a positive way, and not to think of problem areas as "disabilities" (even though they may be diagnosed as such). I like sports analogies, or animal analogies. For sports, I might talk about how a baseball player is a great fielder and hitter, but needs work on this throwing, to make him or her a better player, with the "therapist" seen as a coach. Talking about animals is great because you can emphasize how animals adapt to the world so differently and can be so special, based on what they have been given at birth. Birds who hunt fish solve the problem of fishing by having extraordinary eyesight and strong talons. Turtles who are incredibly slow have a hard shell. Animals especially vulnerable to daytime predators may be nocturnal. Each animal has solved a series of problems which has allowed them to flourish. Each is different but special in its own right.

Children must also learn to learn about and adapt to who they are. We can help nourish their strengths, and bolster their weaknesses. We must help each one find what is unique about his or her spirit.

Action Points

1. If you think your child has learning problems, consult the child's teacher first, and then possibly a learning specialist or psychologist.
2. For developmental delays in speech, fine motor, or gross motor functioning, consult a specialist for an evaluation.
3. For suspected problems with social functioning, ask your child's teachers, coaches, and other mentors for input, and observe how your child interacts with others for more clues.
4. If you see delays in any of these areas (cognitive, fine motor, gross motor, or social functioning), see your pediatrician for help initially.
5. Look for signs of emotionally based problems, such as depression, anxiety, or stress which can also affect development and functioning with friends and in school.
6. Different specialists—psychologists, psychiatrists, neurologists, physical therapists, occupational therapists—can help your child overcome different developmental challenges.

CHAPTER 9

How Your Child Behaves
and Functions

A child's existence is very physical. Most of a child's day is spent running and jumping, moving from place to place, sitting in school, eating and drinking, in short, interfacing with the physical world. This chapter examines how the way children behave affects how they function in the world.

Sleepy Heads

Fourteen-year-old Julie was referred to me because her school performance was failing, she was having problems falling asleep, and her parents were concerned that she seemed negative and moody. This busy ninth grader was a pitcher for her school softball team, a member of the debate team, the organizer of a youth group at her temple, and worked at the temple on Sunday mornings. Often, she was not home until nine at night, and then had to start her schoolwork. "I feel like I have to keep all of this up or it will affect which college I get into," Julie told me.

Clearly, she was under considerable stress, and felt tired during the day, which contributed to her problems falling asleep at night. I suggested to Julie and her parents that by doing everything for a purpose, or because it was expected of her, Julie wasn't paying enough attention to her own health and happiness. I recommended that she sleep in on

Sundays for a few months and not work at the temple to ease some of her stress, and gave her some relaxation exercises to help her fall asleep. I suggested that she see a psychotherapist to help her work through negative feelings about herself and why she felt it was easier to do what others expected of her, rather than what might be best for herself. I mentioned that her sleep loss may be the beginning of depression, which ran in her family, and that we follow any other depressive symptoms quite closely. They all agreed to look at Julie's sleep problem as a signal from her body that something was not right, to work on reducing her stress, and to investigate what role depression might play. Much of this seems like common sense, doesn't it? Yet, when in the thick of it, even the best parents can miss the forest for the trees, and not realize when a child who seems to be able to handle it all is showing signs of wear and tear.

Translation: "Sleep and fatigue are just the tip of the iceberg. I'm overextended and feel that I don't do enough, even though another part of me knows I do too much. But I can't stop."

Sleep problems can disturb a child's social life and academic functioning. But some children may have night terrors or nightmares, or may sleepwalk. Sleep can be affected by ADHD, depression, a medical illness, or even substance abuse.

Examples of the many types of sleep problems, according the American Academy of Child and Adolescent Psychiatry, include: frequent awakenings during the night, talking during sleep, difficulty falling asleep, waking up crying, feeling sleepy during the day, having nightmares, bedwetting, teeth grinding and clenching, and waking early.

One of the most common problems parents face is a child who won't stay in bed. Usually, these younger children haven't yet learned how to put themselves to sleep. The first task is for you to get out of the child's bed. If your child can't tolerate your being out of sight, sit in a chair next to the bed until the child falls asleep. Gradually, physically detach yourself, moving a little closer to the door each night until you are out of the room. Then, take breaks from your child's line of vision, returning to the chair when you say you will. Gradually increase the amount of time you are gone. Parents can get into the habit of lying with their child or stroking them to get them to sleep. This can lead to problems, since the child may not be able to fall asleep any other way, and when they awake during the night, as all children briefly do as they traverse the architecture of sleep, they will need to have their parents in order to fall back asleep.

School-age kids may also have sleep problems when they feel normal childhood anxieties. If the problem has just come up, find out about any conflicts in school or with friends, and try to resolve them. If the problem is chronic, and your child becomes temperamental, anxious, or fearful, then you have to deal with it on a more behavioral level. You can read books, such as Maurice Sendak's *Where the Wild Things Are*, and give the child a flashlight if he or she is afraid of the dark. Or draw pictures of scary things, then put cages around them, and, finally, rip them up and throw them in the garbage, physically and symbolically.

For older children, napping during the day can lead to not sleeping at night. Teens tend to stay up late, become sleep deprived during the week, and make up for it on the weekend. One way to get them back on the sleep track is to set their bedtime back fifteen minutes a night over time, and to set a no-napping policy. Many of you are perhaps laughing at this, realizing that for many teens, this strategy simply will not work. Another way to approach it is to try (desperately, sometimes) to enlist your teen's support in making their hours more human, maybe by appealing to a wish to be healthy and "on top of their game," not only for their academics, but for their sports, and even their social life. I tell my sleepy teens, "You know, you'll be more attractive to others without those dark circles." That sometimes gets them. If not, parents, don't despair too much. They won't be teenagers forever!

Medical conditions may also cause sleep disturbances, from swollen tonsils that obstruct the airway to infections to thyroid problems. For example, obesity can cause insomnia by interfering with breathing during sleep.

Unusual movements seen during sleep may signal a sleep disorder, or a neurological problem, and should be evaluated by a sleep specialist or neurologist. Sleepwalking should be evaluated by such a specialist as well. Sleep terrors are a normal developmental variant in younger children.

Everyone dreams—it's a way for the unconscious mind to work through everyday events. Sometimes those dreams are scary. So an occasional nightmare is normal. Worry only when the same nightmare recurs several times a week, which may be a sign of stress or a traumatic event.

Get a Good Night's Sleep

There is a growing body of scientific evidence showing that inadequate sleep results in tiredness, difficulties with focused attention, irritability, easy frustration, and difficulty modulating impulses and emotions. This is as true for children as it is for adults, although little attention has been paid to the sleep problems of children. Sleep disorders often go unrecognized in children. The symptoms of sleep deprivation may be attributed to hyperactivity, behavior disorders, boredom with school, or to a hectic lifestyle.

To help young children get enough sleep, the National Heart, Lung, and Blood Institute has funded a major five-year educational initiative that targets young children, their parents, teachers, and pediatricians. Their message is that an adequate night's sleep—at least nine hours—will help children do their best in whatever they do, including school, sports, and other extracurricular activities, and will help them maintain good family relationships and friendships. The Institute believes that early intervention with sleep education messages will help children understand the importance of incorporating good sleep habits into their lifestyles early in their lives.

Some school districts are experimenting with another way to help students sleep more—later school starting times, which allow students a chance to catch up on their sleep. While some schools report that high school seniors, in particular, seem to take advantage of a later start, further study is needed to determine if delaying school start times results in improved school performance.

Sleepwalking, Sleep Terrors, and Nightmares (also known as the "Parasomnias")

Sleepwalking tends to run in families, and should be evaluated because the child might get hurt bumping into objects, falling down stairs, or even going outside. Sleepwalking may also include features of sleep terrors, with further risk of injury as your child may strike out, or feel frightened and flee the house. If your child sleepwalks, have him or her evaluated quickly by a sleep specialist. Increasing total sleep time by an hour or so may help. If it doesn't, the condition may be treated with medication.

A sleep specialist can do a sleep recording to help diagnose sleep problems. A sleep recording involves checking the child's brain waves during sleep in an overnight stay at a special sleep lab. An estimated 15 percent of children experience at least one episode of sleepwalking, according to the National Center on Sleep Disorders Research. Sleepwalking usually starts around ages four to eight, peaks at around age twelve, and resolves in adolescence. A fever or sleep deprivation can increase a child's frequency of sleepwalking. If your child has been waking up terrified and screaming at a predictable time after falling asleep, on subsequent nights wake up the child before it happens. Then let your child go back to sleep. At times, this may avert the terror, which usually occurs during the first third of the night. So just before you go to bed, wake your child up to help reset the child's sleep clock.

A child with sleep terror is difficult to wake up or comfort and doesn't remember what happened the next morning. Sleep terror is not to be confused with panic attacks, where your child is afraid and agitated, but fully awake, not confused, and remembers everything about the attack. Sleep terror doesn't mean that your child has psychiatric problems, and generally reflect immaturity of the central nervous system. Sleep terror episodes occur in only a small percentage of children, usually beginning between the ages of four and twelve and resolving spontaneously during adolescence.

Sleep terrors are different than nightmares. During nightmares, the child awakens easily and completely, and remembers the dream. Nightmares usually occur later in the night, with less arousal and irritation, and the child's dream recall is much better than during sleep terror. A recurrent nightmare, or nightmares almost every night, should be looked into, particularly for children who have nightmares following a traumatic event. Some children wake up repeatedly during the night, and recall vivid details of their frightening dreams, which often include threats to their survival or self-esteem. Nightmares occur as part of other mental disorders, such as posttraumatic stress disorder and mood and anxiety disorders. If nightmares occur after a trauma, or occur frequently and affect a child's daytime life, it's time to get help.

As the American Academy of Child and Adolescent Psychiatry notes, parasomnias are not that uncommon in children. However, when they are occurring several times per night, or nightly for a few weeks, or affect a child's functioning during the day, they should be evaluated.

Long Sleepers

Some children need more than normal amounts of sleep, which is called hypersomnia. They sleep ten to twelve hours each night and still can't get up in the morning. They usually are not sleepy during the day. Others may sleep eight hours and take naps during the day. This problem usually begins at around age fifteen and continues into adulthood.

Both insomnia and hypersomnia can relate to other mental disorders, and sleep disorders can relate to medical conditions. Most medical conditions cause a child to get less sleep and to stay awake longer. If your child is having trouble sleeping, you have to figure out whether it is a primary sleep problem, related to a psychiatric problem, or a medical condition.

In narcolepsy, children and adolescents report an increased need for sleep, and may fall asleep during the day spontaneously even after a solid night's sleep. Narcolepsy may be combined with cataplexy, which is the sudden intrusion of rapid eye movement, or dream sleep, into the waking state. This causes sudden fainting, usually during intense emotional arousal, such as anger or surprise. A cataplectic person can see, hear, and feel, but other muscles may be paralyzed. Pediatric sleep expert Ronald Dahl, M.D., reports that asking a cataplectic person to move the eyes to the side three times, or to take some deep breaths, can indicate that a "fainting" spell actually is cataplexy, not a conversion disorder. About half of the time, there is a family history of narcolepsy, with or without cataplexy.

Allergic to Sleep?

During allergy seasons, a child's allergies can cause sleep problems, particularly in falling asleep. Treatment with an oral antihistamine, nasal drops, or eye drops should help clear up the allergy symptoms and allow the child to fall asleep. It's also important to look for potential sources of allergens, or allergy-causing substances, in the bedroom and the house, including dust mites and animal dander. An allergist may recommend that parents remove all rugs (and even pets) from the house, and that all sheets be washed regularly with special detergents that kill dust mites.

Attention Deficit Hyperactivity Disorder

The diagnosis and treatment of attention deficit hyperactivity disorder (ADHD) has sparked a national debate, with many critics questioning the use of drugs to treat young children for symptoms that may be unrelated to the disorder. People with ADHD have persistent problems paying attention and/or controlling their impulses and hyperactivity. Since most children behave this way some of the time, making the diagnosis can be difficult.

Despite all the controversy of who is or isn't hyperactive, there is a well-defined ADHD syndrome of—developmentally inappropriate impulsive behavior, inattentiveness, and hyperactivity seen in multiple settings that begins before age seven. A combination of genetic, imaging, and epidemiological studies show that ADHD is a genuine, neurologically based syndrome. ADHD symptoms can exist into adolescence; these children are susceptible to drug abuse. About three boys are diagnosed to every one girl.

Adhering strictly to the diagnostic criteria as part of a thorough evaluation minimizes both the under- and overdiagnosis of ADHD. ADHD diagnoses have increased because parents and educators are more aware of the disorder. More children with an inattentive variation who are not hyperactive are now being picked up. ADHD is also being identified more often in teens and girls who might not have been diagnosed before, and children are being treated for longer periods of time since it has become more apparent that ADHD is often a chronic problem. Yet, the overall percentage of children being treated with medication who have the disorder is roughly the same.

If your child is diagnosed with ADHD, make sure strict assessment criteria have been used. I spend two hours with a family, as well as time with the child's teacher, and have parents and teachers fill out rating scales. While Ritalin-like drugs are often prescribed, other nondrug treatments can be effective, including changes in the child's environment (including modifications in school), working with the child to help control behaviors, and group counseling that addresses social skills.

ADHD may be seen through the teen years, and in some cases continues into adulthood. Despite these teens' best intentions, cooperating may be difficult. They may be restless, though I've found that oftentimes they are not as hyperactive as little children are. These older ADHD children seem to be always on the go, and may complain of being bored, and may be impulsive when it comes to behavior that could get them in trouble. They may get involved in substance abuse, and tend to have more car accidents.

Some ADHD children aren't diagnosed because their behavior is not disruptive; they don't single themselves out. Children with the ADHD, inattentive subtype, who are bright enough to get passing grades are often overlooked, even though they usually are underachieving. Other ADHD children who go unidentified may have behavioral problems that may be chalked up to "boys being boys." They may willfully not listen, or they don't want to listen. The most famous line I've heard from parents is, "If he wanted to pay attention, he could. If something interests him, he's just fine."

The problem with ADHD is not necessarily that the child can't pay attention—he can't pay attention to something that doesn't interest him. These children may be unable to filter out the extraneous stuff that's all around us. At one point in our ancestry, paying attention to multiple stimuli at once (such as in a threatening environment with many predators), may have been adaptive, acting impulsively may have been more protective than delayed response (for example, if attacked), and motor hyperactivity might have made it easier to find food when it was scarce, according to Columbia's Peter Jensen, M.D., and colleagues. Some of us may have held onto this particular style of dealing with the environment, which does not work well in the classroom.

We all filter out distracting, stimulating information in the world around us. The question is, once we start filtering, how long do we stick with it? That takes persistence, and some ADHD children don't have the wherewithal to do that. A child with ADHD may be able to pay attention to something interesting. But just because a child can watch television or play with a Game Boy for hours on end doesn't mean he can sit and do his math homework. In order to pay attention, one's focus must first be captured; it then must filter out other less important stuff, and it must be able to persist long enough to finish the job.

ADHD and Oppositional Behavior

Nearly half of ADHD children have oppositional defiant disorder (ODD), which is characterized by stubborn behavior, outbursts of temper, belligerence, and defiance. These behaviors significantly affect functioning for these children, in school, home, and with friends. ODD children often lose their temper, argue with adults, and are at risk for getting into trouble at school and with their parents, because they often do not listen to what they are told to do. Research also shows that as early as kindergarten, those children who display hyperactivity and oppositional behavior are more likely to become physically violent when they are older. According to the American Academy of Child and Adolescent Psychiatry, about 5 to 15 percent of children have ODD, with the cause not known, though both biology, and a child's environment, are thought to be important. These children should be evaluated from an early age, since many of them will have other problems, such as ADHD, conduct disorder, mood disorders, and learning disabilities. We can do a lot to help these kids and their families, including parent training (no parent is born knowing how to deal with ODD children effectively, believe me, and the sense of failure and frustration I often see is so unfair to the parents), anger management training for the kids, and social skills groups to help these kids learn how to make friends and keep them. Working with these kids individually can help teach them how to manage problems in a positive way. In their "Facts for Families" series, the Child Academy offers the following suggestions:

- Always build on the positives, give the child praise and positive reinforcement when he shows flexibility or cooperation.
- Take a time-out or break if you are about to make the conflict with your child worse, not better. This is good modeling for your child. Support your child if she decides to take a time-out to prevent overreacting.
- Pick your battles. Since the child with ODD has trouble avoiding power struggles, prioritize the things you want your child to do. If you give your child a time-out in his room for misbehavior, don't add time for arguing. Say "your time will start when you go to your room."
- Set up reasonable, age appropriate limits with consequences that can be enforced consistently.
- Maintain interests other than your child with ODD, so that managing your child doesn't take all your time and energy. Try to work with and obtain support from the other adults (teachers, coaches, and spouse) dealing with your child.
- Manage your own stress with exercise and relaxation. Use respite care as needed.

ADHD and Other Disorders

What looks like ADHD may be something that goes along with the disorder. According to Children and Adults with Attention-Deficit/Hyperactivity Disorder (CHADD), a national self-help group for ADHD, ADHD can occur with learning disabilities (15 to 25 percent), language disorders (30 to 35 percent), and tic disorders (up to 60 percent). About 25 percent of children with ADHD have an anxiety disorder, which can worsen their attention problems. About 20 percent have mood disorders, which can also make them feel down or moody, and affect sleep, appetite, friendships and school. From 15 to 20 percent of ADHD children may develop conduct disorder, which leads them to be aggressive toward people or animals, destroy property, lie or steal, and violate rules, such as being truant from school, not obeying curfews, or running away from home.

Many children with fetal alcohol syndrome show signs of ADHD. Some people believe that cocaine can also lead to ADHD-like behaviors. Sleep disorders are also more prevalent among ADHD children.

Recent Research Findings

Brain imaging research has suggested that the brains of children with ADHD are different. Results from positron emission tomography (PET) have linked a child's inability to pay attention with metabolism in specific areas in the brain. Glucose, or sugar, is the body's major fuel. In adults with ADHD, the brain areas that control attention use less glucose and appear to be less active, suggesting that a lower level of activity in some parts of the brain may cause inattention.

ADHD tends to run in families, so genetics is likely to play a role. ADHD children usually have at least one close relative who also has ADHD. At least one-third of all fathers who had ADHD when they were young have children with ADHD. While food additives were once considered a contributing factor in the disorder, a National Institute of Health study in 1982 concluded that restricted diets help only about 5 percent of those with ADHD, mostly young children or those with allergies. Stimulant medications are the most well studied ADHD treatment. A recent, comprehensive scientific report confirmed many earlier studies showing that short-term use of stimulants is safe and effective for children with ADHD. In December 1999, the National Institute of Mental Health released the first results of a study of nearly 600 elementary school children, ages seven to nine, which evaluated the safety and relative effectiveness of the leading treatments for ADHD for up to fourteen months. The results show that stimulants are more effective than behavioral therapies in controlling the core symptoms of ADHD—inattention, hyperactivity/impulsiveness, and aggression. A combination of stimulants with intensive behavioral therapies was consistently more effective in improving anxiety symptoms, academic performance, and social skills. Interestingly, families and teachers reported somewhat higher levels of satisfaction for treatments that included the behavioral therapy components. So there is certainly room for both drug and behavioral therapy in the treatment of ADHD. For more about treating ADHD, see Chapter 16.

Another randomized study of teens with ADHD has shown that drug therapy with methylphenidate (Ritalin) may relieve both behavioral symptoms and learning difficulties better than a placebo. The forty-five teens participated in an eight-week intensive summer treatment program at the University of Pittsburgh. They attended a history class four days a week and participated in other activities that helped them with note taking, social skills, and problem solving. Their parents received training in behavior management techniques.

Every day, the teens received one of three different doses of the drug or a placebo. On days that they were taking the drug, about 80 percent of the teens improved their note-taking quality, quiz and work sheet scores, written language, homework completion, and behavior. Two-thirds showed the greatest improvement while on the lowest dose (10 milligrams). Half of the remaining teens improved with the 20-milligram dose, and very few improved with a 30-milligram dose.

This is the first large study to show that methylphenidate can improve school performance in teenagers with ADHD. The results need to be verified in a larger group, and the effects of the drug need to be established over a longer period of time. But parents who are considering drug therapy for a teen with ADHD may find improvement in school performance in addition to social skills.

The Multimodal Treatment of ADHD (MTA) study, a large multicenter treatment study, will be discussed in Chapter 16.

Bullies

Bullying has become a hotly debated topic in the media as a result of the seemingly increasing numbers of gun violence incidents in schools. Bullies generally have been bullied by someone else, and have problems of their own. Anger management programs can help them control their anger and aggression.

Surveys indicate that as many as half of all children are bullied, either physically or verbally, at some time during their school years, and at least 10 percent are bullied on a regular basis, according to the Child Academy. A National Institute of Child Health and Human Development (NICHHD) study led by Tonja Nansel, Ph.D., confirmed that the prevalence of bullying among American youth is substantial. Almost 30 percent of the nearly 16,000 students from both public and private schools in sixth to tenth grade said they were moderately or frequently involved in bullying. Many younger children hide throughout the school day. As they grow older, they are more likely to take more active measures to protect themselves. Some will begin to carry a weapon to school; others will become part of a gang for protection. Still others will simply drop out of school.

The NICHHD study also found that boys bully more than girls, and middle school children more than teens. Boys tend to bully with physical and verbal threats, while girls more often use verbal bullying such as name calling, spreading rumors, and teasing. In this age of computers, bullying has even been reported in online chatrooms and through e-mail.

As the NICHHD study found, both bullies and those who are bullied are likely to suffer problems with social and emotional development and in school performance. Bullies tend to have conduct problems and don't like school; those who are bullied generally seem more insecure, anxious, depressed, lonely, unhappy, and have low self-esteem. Some victims of bullying have even attempted suicide rather than endure the harassment and punishment. Others attempt to strike back at society through violent acts.

Bullies thrive on domination. They often have been physically abused or bullied themselves, and may also be depressed, angry, or upset about how things are going at school or at home. Bullies often pick on children who are passive, easily intimidated, or have few friends. Often, their victims are smaller or younger, and can't defend themselves easily.

If you suspect your child is bullying others, it's important to seek help as soon as possible from your child's pediatrician, teacher, principal, or school counselor. Continued bullying behavior may lead to serious academic, social, emotional, and legal difficulties. If necessary, arrange for a child psychiatrist or other mental health professional to conduct a comprehensive evaluation. The evaluation should help you and your child understand why he or she is a bully, and help you develop a plan to stop the behavior.

If you suspect your child may be the victim of bullying, talk to your child in an open, honest way about what's happening. Let your child know it's not his or her fault, and that he or she did the right thing by telling you. Together, brainstorm about what you think you should do. Find out what your child has already tried, and whether it helped or not.

Most bullying goes on at school—in the playground, lunchroom, bathrooms, or hallway between classes, or on the school bus. Ask your child's teacher or the school guidance counselor for more feedback on the situation at school. Find out about programs your child's school or community may have to help suppress bullying. These programs may include peer mediation, conflict resolution, and anger management training, as well as increased adult supervision. In fact, schools MUST take a central role in dealing with bullying. Working with a bullied child, without substantial change occurring in the environment to protect the child, will not change much.

Researchers from the LaMarsh Centre on Violence and Conflict Resolution in Toronto used covert videotaping to study bullying behavior. They found that on average, four peers viewed the schoolyard bullying, with a range from two to fourteen peers. Peers spent 54 percent of their time reinforcing bullies by passively watching, 21 percent of their time actively modeling after the bullies, and 25 percent of their time intervening on behalf of victims. Older boys (grades 4–6) were more likely to actively join with the bully than were younger boys (grades 1–3) and older girls. Both younger and older girls were more likely to intervene on behalf of victims than were older boys. These results underscore the central role of peers in playground bullying episodes. Peers' antibullying initiatives must be accompanied by simultaneous whole-school interventions.

Eating Problems

School-age children can be finicky eaters. Unless they are truly sick, they usually will eat enough, so don't become preoccupied if your children don't take in enough calories in any one day. What's more important is how they fit on standard growth curves. If your child falls off the curve or stops gaining weight, then it's time to investigate. Abdominal pain and persistent vomiting can cause a failure to gain weight. While parents will never win a battle to "force" their children to eat more healthy foods, having less high-calorie, fatty foods around the house, and setting an example by eating healthy foods, can help children develop better eating habits. Having your children accompany you to the supermarket to help "choose" more healthy foods can sometimes help, or making "deals" with your children to try one new "healthy" food per week, to see if they like it. They may surprise themselves, and you. Such was the case recently in an Italian restaurant when all four of my kids announced they wanted some of the salad my wife and I ordered, because it looked so appetizing, and the oil and vinegar dressing was just right.

Eating disorders are uncommon until adolescence, and are more common among girls. A national screening of high school students for eating disorders has found that nearly one-third of girls and 16 percent of boys show symptoms of an eating disorder. Anorexia nervosa, the voluntary restriction of food intake associated with a distorted body image causing substantial weight loss, and bulimia nervosa, the binge-and-purge syndrome, are caused by distorted body image. Fighting over food consumption is a common first response by parents, but usually gets you nowhere. Some signs of anorexia nervosa include a teenage girl who has lost so much weight that she stops menstruating, abuses laxatives, diet pills, or diuretics, and exercises compulsively. These eating disorders require a psychological evaluation.

Anorexia and Bulimia

Anorexia is characterized by extreme weight loss, and is generally defined as a child who is at least 15 percent below normal body weight. Although many children with the disorder become emaciated, they believe that they are overweight. The child refuses to eat due to a fear of getting fat, which usually derives from a distorted body image. In other words, these girls look in the mirror and feel overweight, or that certain body parts are too large, even though they are very thin. Sometime, they starve themselves to the point of needing hospitalization. About 1 percent of all women have anorexia.

The anorexic's obsession with food and weight may lead to compulsive or bizarre food habits, such as cutting food into tiny pieces and counting bites, or refusing to eat in front of people. Some also stick to stringent exercise routines. It is important to rule out the existence of another psychiatric disorder, such as obsessive-compulsive disorder (OCD), social phobia, or body dysmorphic disorder (BDD).

The medical complications of anorexia include the loss of menstrual periods, lowered blood pressure and pulse, slowed thyroid function, brittle hair and nails, constipation, reduced tolerance to cold temperatures, anemia, swollen joints, reduced muscle mass, and lightheadedness. In serious cases, starvation damages vital organs, including the brain and heart. Calcium loss from bones may make them brittle and prone to fracture.

Bulimia is characterized by binging—consuming large amounts of food—and then purging—ridding the body of food, nutrients, and calories by vomiting, abusing laxatives, using diuretics or enemas, or exercising excessively. Bulimics eat ridiculously large amounts of food in a very short time and then may purge out of a sense of guilt. According to B. Timothy Walsh, M.D., about half of anorexics have the binge/purge subtype. He believes that the frequency of this subtype tends to increase with the duration of illness, so probably much fewer teen anorexics have the binge/purge subtype.

The definition of bulimia excludes anorexia, so no one with a current diagnosis of bulimia can have anorexia. The real distinction is weight: bulimics are, almost always, of normal weight. About one-third of bulimics have past histories of anorexia. From 1 to 3 percent of young adolescents, mostly girls, have bulimia.

The medical complications from bulimia include tooth decay, inflammation of the esophagus, and swollen glands.

Fortunately, eating disorders can be treated. Early detection and diagnosis is key. Because a complex interaction of physical, psychological, and emotional components is involved, a team of experts is usually involved, including physicians, nutritionists, psychotherapists, and psychopharmacologists.

Antidepresssants appear to reduce purging, even if the person is not depressed. Individual, group, and family therapies are also useful. A wide network of national and local resources is available to help children with eating disorders and their families.

Other Eating Problems

In addition to anorexia and bulimia, general medical conditions can cause serious weight loss, including gastrointestinal diseases and tumors. Psychiatric disorders, such as depression, can cause weight loss as well. Children with OCD or certain pervasive developmental disorder can also have food compulsions. Those with sensory integration problems may have issues with food texture—they don't like things that are crunchy or chewy. Eating nonfoods such as paint, plaster, string, hair, cloth, sand, insects, leaves, pebbles, and clay can be associated with pervasive developmental disorders and mental retardation. Lastly, bona fide food allergies can affect food intake. For example, allergy to birch pollen may cause a child to have an itchy sensation in his mouth when he eats peaches or strawberries.

Drug and Alcohol Abuse

Drugs and alcohol continue to be a persistent problem among today's teens. If you suspect your child is using drugs, first get information on the child's functioning.

Some of the warning signs of substance abuse include complaints about feeling tired, having red, glassy eyes, and coughing persistently; a personality change, including sudden mood swings, feeling irritable or depressed, acting irresponsibly, having low self-esteem, and exercising poor judgment; instigating arguments, breaking rules, or withdrawing from family life; having little interest in school, a drop in grades, regularly being absent or late to school, and having discipline problems; making new friends who couldn't care less about home and school activities, having problems with the police. Obviously, depression can cause some of the same symptoms, as can simply being a teenager. Don't forget that substance abuse not uncommonly goes along with depression in teens who are medicating themselves with illicit substances to feel better.

Obviously, some of these symptoms can be caused by other problems, such as depression, or other things that might be stressing your adolescent. To start, ask your pediatrician to talk to your child during a routine exam. A confirmed diagnosis rests on a urine sample. However, only fat soluble drugs such as marijuana tend to hang out long enough in the body to cause a positive toxicology screen several days after using it, and this also depends on how much the teen has been smoking and for how long. Other drugs leave the body too quickly to pick up unless the toxicology screen is done close to the time of drug usage. Teens who use drugs are often up on ways to disguise a toxicology screen, as well, by adding water, substituting urine samples, or adding substances to the urine.

Sometimes teens do drugs or alcohol to self-medicate anxiety problems or depression. They may be curious, want to "feel good," be more like an adult, or be part of a group. They may also feel stress at home, and act out as a way to get attention. If family issues and conflicts are part of the drug or alcohol abuse, then they have to be dealt with as well.

Some teens experiment with drugs and alcohol, and stop, or use them only occasionally without significant problems. Others, however, may develop a dependency, and move on to more dangerous drugs. Teens may be more at risk for developing serious drug or alcohol problems if they have a family history of substance abuse, are depressed, have low self-esteem and feel they don't fit in.

The use of illegal drugs is increasing, especially among young teens. Marijuana and alcohol are commonly used by today's high school students. The most commonly used illegal drugs are marijuana; stimulants such as cocaine, crack, and speed; hallucinogens such as LSD and PCP; narcotics such as opiates and heroin; and designer drugs, mainly Ecstasy ("E"), or ketamine ("K"). Legally available drugs include alcohol; prescription medications such as pain killers; inhalants such as glues, aerosols, and solvents; and over-the-counter cough, cold, sleep, and diet drugs.

Drug and alcohol users are at increased risk of using serious drugs later in life. They may fail at school, and their poor judgment may lead them into accidents, violence, unplanned and unsafe sex, and even suicide. Teens who are abusing drugs or alcohol generally need to be in a substance abuse treatment program. If they are addicted, they need to be "detoxed" first in an inpatient unit, and then transitioned into an intensive outpatient program.

Parents can help prevent drug or alcohol abuse by talking about the issue openly, early, and often. Good communication and early recognition of potential problems are the keys. Early education in schools is also essential, as well as community-based programs and advertising campaigns, such as those directed at drunk driving.

While parents may recognize the signs of potential abuse, they shouldn't be expected to make the diagnosis. If your adolescent has some of the signs listed above, don't immediately jump to suspect substance abuse. Give your child the benefit of the doubt, and look for other problems, such as depression or stress. You can show you care by openly discussing drug and alcohol abuse with your child. Get help, if necessary.

Action Plan

For sleep problems, take an inventory and define the problem by answering the following questions: How many hours does your child sleep at night? When does your child go to bed? fall asleep? wake up? What does your child do in the hour before bedtime? Does your child have a television in the bedroom? Does the child fall asleep with the radio on? Electronic devices are often stimulating, and though as adults we may be used to falling asleep with the TV on, this is often not the case with children. Does your child have a regular sleep schedule? Can the child fall asleep on his or her own?

Good sleep hygiene is a must for a child with sleep problems. Try to have a regular bedtime. For a preschool or school-age child, parents should set the bedtime. For adolescents, negotiate. Try to have regular bedtime rituals. In our house, it's bath, brush and floss teeth, and read a book—the older girls read to themselves, and either my wife or I read to the younger ones. Keep in mind that if teens go to sleep regularly after midnight, they essentially have a "sleep phase shift" problem (i.e., it's as if they are living in another time zone). When they crash out on the weekends to catch up, and awaken at 12 P.M. or later, they reinforce this phase shift, making it harder to get to sleep earlier during the week. A commitment by the adolescent to change this pattern is essential, and involves gradually moving back to a "normal" time zone.

I suggest you have no stimulating activities in the hour before bedtime, including computer and television. I find it's better to be read to or to read a book. Children who feel too wound up before bedtime may benefit from imagery, breathing exercises, muscle relaxation, or reading a book—but no ghost stories or thrillers. Some children also benefit from having a night-light.

For preschool children who are having difficulty sleeping, I suggest reading stories or using imagery before they go to sleep. Tell your child: Imagine that you're a rag doll or a wet noodle, or that you are like Jell-O. Have them imagine they are in a comfy, warm, safe place and can enter dreamland.

For older children, my Columbia University colleague, Candace Erickson, M.D., suggests this relaxation technique before bedtime. Invite your child as follows: You may want to take a deep breathe in and as you let it out slowly, you can imagine a special place. Perhaps it's the beach, or the park, or anywhere you like—a place where you are safe, comfortable, and relaxed—and you just allow your imagination to take you to that place. You can notice what it feels like when you're there . . . I wonder what you see . . . Perhaps there are smells . . . I wonder what you hear . . . You can use as many of your senses as you like as you become more relaxed and comfortable. You can slowly breathe in deeply through your nose and then slowly breathe out comfortably through your mouth. As you breathe in, you may want to imagine that you are filling up a balloon in your tummy. And as you breathe out, you can just let go of the air from your lungs. And you can just continue relaxing with your breathing as you enjoy being in the special place.

If your child has insomnia, that is, wakes up in the middle of the night and can't fall back asleep, take a week or two to figure out what might be causing it. If it continues for longer than two weeks, see your pediatrician. A preschooler's sleep terrors that last for a week or two may be a normal part of development. However, a few weeks of sleep terrors in older children could be the sign of a neurological problem, and should be evaluated by a neurologist. Similarly, if your teenager oversleeps for more than two weeks, have your pediatrician conduct a check up.

If your child is not getting enough sleep, or needs more than an average amount of sleep, try to regularize the child's sleep cycle. If your child gets less than seven hours of sleep at night, put together a regular sleep hygiene program. If your child sleeps more than nine hours a night and falls asleep during the day, think about other causes, including substance abuse or depression, or even narcolepsy.

When dealing with ADHD, insist on a comprehensive evaluation. About 75 percent of the time some other problem accompanies ADHD that must also be addressed. Included in the evaluation should be a careful review of your child's symptoms, a medical evaluation, and a lab workup. Many children with suspected ADHD don't routinely get blood tests, but an overactive thyroid can lead to some similar symptoms. Also, the side effects of asthma medication can mimic ADHD symptoms.

To evaluate your child's learning and cognitive skills, you should get information from multiple sources. Yes, you see your child at home, but how does he or she do at school and after school? To be diagnosed with ADHD a child should have symptoms in at least two settings. So, a child who is a pain in the neck at home and does fine in school may not be diagnosed as ADHD. Psychiatrists look for really clear evidence of impairment in social, academic, or family functioning that significantly affects your child. A very bright child in an understimulating academic environment may be inattentive as well. A psychiatrist may also ask about your child's vision and hearing, and any history of seizures, allergies, or nutrition problems. For example, caffeine in soft drinks may also make a child seem hyperactive. The doctor will gather the information from the interviews about your child's behavior and his or her teacher's observations to try to make an accurate diagnosis.

Your pediatrician can make the diagnosis if a child psychiatrist is unavailable, but it's a challenge. The pediatrician will have to collect information from multiple sources, and interview your child and you, which could take several visits. Your child will need a medical evaluation by the pediatrician, and possibly specialists such as a neurologist.

Confounding factors may get in the way of the diagnosis. A child who has had a recent trauma—a death in the family, or even a chronic ear infection—can become uncooperative. Other such factors include living with family members who are physically abusive or who abuse alcohol or drugs or a learning disability that makes schoolwork too hard and leaves a child not developmentally ready to read or write. All facets of your child's life have to be considered to understand their impact on your child's development.

Educational options are available for ADHD children, including preferential seating, extra time on tests, and assignments written on the blackboard. A written list of rules and rewards for good behavior may also help. Some educational materials may help as well. Mel Levine's *A Mind at a Time* is a terrific book about learning differences in children, as is *The Misunderstood Child: Understanding and Coping with Your Child's Learning Disabilities* by Larry B. Silver. Excellent books about ADHD and ODD include: *Dr. Larry Silver's Advice to Parents on Attention Deficit Hyperactivity Disorder,* by Larry B. Silver; *Taking Charge of ADHD,* Revised Edition, and *Your Defiant Child,* both by Russell A. Barkley. Teachers may provide school assignments on a computer for children who have trouble writing them down. And school districts in affluent communities have been know to provide Palm Pilots for some ADHD children.

A special education teacher can devise an individualized educational program for your child. Every child has the right to receive special programs under the federal Individuals with Disabilities Education Act.

Children with ADHD have extremely short attention spans and have difficulty following complex directions. That's why it's important to break tasks down into very small bits. If your child has twenty-five mathematics problems, ask him or her to do five at a time throughout the evening until the homework is completed. In addition, when you give your child instructions, keep them short and simple. Directions longer than one sentence may be too long.

The basic message remains to get a good evaluation, don't blame your child for "acting up," and try to remove any misconceptions about what treatment should be. Have an open mind. The best treatment for ADHD often combines educational and behavioral approaches, with or without medication.

If your child is being bullied, first ensure your child's safety. You don't want your child to be aggressive, but you can teach ways to respond that don't get your child into trouble. Walking away sometimes works, but a verbal comeback often can put a bully in his or her place. You and your child can practice being assertive and come up with something to say to the bully so that your child is ready for the next encounter. Just saying "Leave me alone!" and walking away may be enough. I also suggest that your child travel with friends back and forth to school, during shopping trips, or on other outings. Bullies are less likely to pick on a child in a group. If you do confront the bully's parents, do it in person and in a calm and nonthreatening manner. Remember that without a systemic approach to dealing with bullies, just working with a child who is bullied will fail. Parents need to be assertive about having the school deal with the bullying problem.

If your child becomes withdrawn, depressed, or reluctant to go to school, or if you see a decline in school performance, speak with the principal, or even the superintendent if the matter is not dealt with satisfactorily and is occurring in school. A child might also benefit from a consultation with a mental health professional. With the professional's help, your and your child and the school can develop a strategy to deal with the bullying, and lessen the risk of lasting emotional scars.

A growing number of schools across the country have adopted bully-proofing programs in an attempt to change attitudes so that bullying is no longer tolerated. Some liken it to the issue of drunk driving. We used to accept this as a minor offense until groups like Mothers Against Drunk Driving and Students Against Drunk Driving convinced people of the horrors of drunk driving, and helped change attitudes. School-based mental health programs can intervene in bullying and help catch problems that could lead to aggression or suicide. Teachers' manuals offer teachers tips on how to intervene with bullies and teach children problem-solving techniques and anger management skills. If your child's school has such a program, ask for the research that shows that it works. There are programs that may be ineffective, or even make matters worse.

For eating disorders, I want to emphasize that finicky eaters are not necessarily anorexics or more likely to become anorexic. Make sure to have healthy food around the house. One solid meal a day is often enough for a young child. The main issue is weight, not what you see your child eat. If your child is gaining weight along his or her "growth curve," I wouldn't worry too much.

Don't get into power struggles with your child over food. It's not necessary to micromanage food every day. Provide a healthy diet and monitor how much your child eats. But use weight gain as a guide, instead of how much your child eats. Checking your child's growth curve periodically, when you visit your pediatrician, is better than putting your child on a scale every week.

If you suspect that your child has a drug or alcohol abuse problem, have your child evaluated medically first. Your pediatrician can refer you to a specialist familiar with drug or alcohol abuse. If your suspicions are confirmed, your child will likely need to attend either an outpatient or inpatient drug or alcohol abuse program, depending on the severity of the problem. It's a mistake to think that once-a-week psychotherapy will cure drug or alcohol abuse. Well-run substance abuse programs include regular toxicology screens to make sure that your child is drug-free or alcohol-free. Some programs run for sixty to ninety days, followed by referral to a twelve-step program, such as Narcotics Anonymous or Alcoholics Anonymous. Some residential inpatient programs las tone year or more.

You want to ascertain whether your child needs to be detoxed, that is, needs to get all of the drugs or alcohol out of his or her body. This step is important because some addicts will undergo withdrawal if they suddenly stop using, depending on the drug being abused. Ask your pediatrician or the drug or alcohol abuse specialist about how to help your child go through detoxification.

Action Points

1. Put together a good sleep hygiene program, including relaxation techniques, if necessary.
2. Make sure to get a comprehensive evaluation before labeling your child as ADHD. The best treatment often combines educational, behavioral, and medical components.

3. Teach your child to be assertive in the face of bullies. Get help from your child's school and, if need be, mental health professionals.
4. Keep healthy food in the house, but don't have daily fights over what your child eats. If you suspect an eating disorder, have a pediatric evaluation, as well as a psychological or psychiatric evaluation.
5. If your child is abusing drugs or alcohol, get help from your pediatrician and specialized programs.

CHAPTER 10

How Your Child Relates to School and Home Environments

*J*ohn, a thirteen-year-old, began ninth grade seemingly without any problems, but then he mysteriously began to miss days of school, complaining of vague ailments. John denied feeling depressed or anxious, and said he simply didn't know why he couldn't get himself to go to school. In fact, though he might actually get up and shower in the morning, he would never make it out of the house. His parents felt he was just faking it, because he was lazy. Actually, John was quite upset and concerned about his inability to get himself to go to school. His parents were quite angry with John, and were at a loss for what to do since he was too big to force to go to school. His school principal took a hard line, saying that he would not tolerate any further absences.

I found out that John had seemed to get by in past years without studying much because he was bright. Suddenly, he found himself in a high-powered high school, and found it hard to keep up. John also admitted that he was anxious being around new classmates. He found himself eating alone at lunch, and generally feeling quite self-conscious. Together we told his parents about his problem, and got him additional academic support from a tutor. He also attended regular meetings with a guidance counselor who ran a peer group for students. John returned to school and after an extremely stressful first day, full of headaches and stomachaches and multiple phone calls to his father, things seemed to settle down. He pulled straight B's for the quarter, made a couple of friends, and was on his way.

Translation: "I'm not lazy. I don't want to go to school because I'm nervous about being in school."

As children get older, they spend less time with their parents, and they like to report less to their parents as a way of separating and showing their independence. Often, they won't report things to avoid disappointing their parents, or to avoid getting teased about Mom and Dad getting involved in their affairs. Add in after-school activities, and children spend as much time away from as with their parents. This chapter looks at how the school and home environment affect your child's life.

Real Quality Time

Today's busy parents have to interface with multiple people and organizations, all of which take time away from being with their children. With all that's going on, it's easy to fool yourself into thinking that taking your children on an errand is spending quality time with them. I suggest that parents do what I recommend for all young doctors: sign out the beeper and leave your cell phone off. A call on a cell phone can interrupt even the quietest moments, and you leave yourself open to easy access if you carry a cell phone. The *Rugrats* cartoon parodies this with Angelica's mother, Charlotte, who's constantly on the cell phone, talking to her personal assistant Jonathan. If you can't turn the phone off, at least set aside some regular time to be with your children without any interruptions. A parent's undivided attention nurtures a child. Like the sun and rain nurture a growing flower, your attention provides your child with the necessary environment to blossom.

No, Really, I'm Okay

Don't be misled by superficial denial, on your part or on the part of your child. It's easy for parents to convince themselves that it's all right to physically be with a child, but not to be there emotionally. Children are adaptable and can get used to their parents not being there for them without realizing how negatively this affects them. They may not complain about a parent's emotional absence, out of fear of upsetting the parent. A teenager whose parents recently split up put it succinctly: "Why bother being upset about something I can't change?"

Children also use denial as a major coping strategy. They often consciously deny being affected by the stresses of life—yet they are affected. School-age children, in particular, can mislead their parents into believing that everything's all right when it isn't. If a child consciously denies stress during stressful times—a move to a new home or school or a sibling getting sick—look at how the child is behaving at that time, not just what she or he is saying. I often tell children that sometimes our bodies react when we're stressed before our minds do, so that the tummyaches and headaches may be a "signal" that something is bothering the child.

Environmental Influences

Behavioral changes can also be brought on by the child's environment. For example, if your child is hyperactive, before assuming it relates to the child's relationships or that it's inherited, consider the elements of your child's diet, any medication she or he is taking, or other things, such as paint chips, she or he may be ingesting:

A diet filled with sugary, chocolate-riddled junk food can make some children so jumpy they seem hyperactive. Hyperactivity could also be a side effect of medication for an asthmatic child, and affect the child's activity level. Check your home for lead-based paint, since eating lead-based paint chips can make a child hyperactive, as can inhaling dust containing lead from household renovations. An intravenously drawn lead level is much more accurate then a finger stick, when lead is measured. Think of your child's entire world and all of the daily interactions with the environment before you jump to any conclusions about symptoms.

School Daze

Just as most parents interact with many people during a typical work day, children meet and greet many people at school, including their friends, teachers, school administrators, and coaches. Parents may be completely unaware of much that goes on in a child's world. And children share little of what goes on, depending on the mood they are in. Even if they are in the right mood, they may leave out details.

In our house, we let each child have the floor for a few minutes each night to talk about his or her day without interruptions from the other children. We encourage them to talk about whatever they want to, with some prompting about what happened that was fun, what they learned, what they did with their friends. If you ask leading questions, be specific rather than asking general questions like "How was your day?" Kids feel better dealing with specifics. For example, ask, "How was the walk and/or ride to school?" "Did you go outside during recess?" "What was for lunch?" "Do you like your teacher? What does she look like? Is she funny?" "Did you get homework? Is it hard? Can I help you with it?" Try to imagine yourself going through your child's day. Also, think of the things you remember doing in school and use that as a guide to ask questions.

When your children answer, give them your full attention. But don't push if they don't want to talk. This shouldn't be like pulling teeth.

You should also take advantage of Back-to-School nights and parent-teacher conferences. There's no substitute for being there at school to find out what's really going on. If you can, drop your child off and pick your child up from school and see how the child looks and interacts with friends. Parent-teacher conferences allow you to see what your child is actually doing in class and affords you the opportunity to talk to your child's teacher about any concerns you or your child may have.

Don't Take Me So Literally

When my seven-year-old son Zach started first grade, I asked him how school was going, and he said "fine" every night for the first week. Then, as I was putting him to bed before the second week of school, Zach blurted out, "No one likes me." I knew that the paperwork piled on my desk would have to wait. We talked about how he might have misconceived how his classmates felt about him. Together, we came up with ways to engage the other children in activities with him, and I told him that either my wife or I would talk to his teacher about it. His teacher, said that Zach was getting along quite well with his classmates. His comment reflected his general anxiety about being in the first grade. A couple of weeks later, after he'd had a few play dates with classmates, Zach again said things were fine, and they really were.

Translation: "I'm afraid that other kids won't like me. In my mind, it's already true."

Children often make specific comments about things that reflect general issues, but don't know how to express themselves. They may say that "school stinks," when they mean that they had an upsetting conversation with the teacher, or did poorly on a quiz. So, sometimes specific complaints can reflect other issues that a child has a difficult time talking about.

So how do you figure this out? Do a little investigating about the child's complaint and what's on the child's mind. If you can't confirm it was the specific issue raised, then look for other more general causes. The complaint may be a signal that something is up and needs some attention. For example, sometimes a child might say that he is "bored" when he really is tired or hungry.

Listen carefully to the child's tone and let the child rest or eat before going on a tear finding things for him or her to do. And don't get too focused on proving or disproving the specific complaint. Sometimes children will present something they fear will become real. Rather than get into the issue of disproving the child's comment, think about how the child may be expressing a concern or masking something else that's harder to talk about.

Action Plan

Take a look at how much time you're spending with your children. Think about how much attention you pay them compared to the rest of your life. You can make minor changes in the amount of attention you pay to them and their emotional issues without impacting on your own ability to function. Ask yourself honestly how things are flowing at home. Life can be frenetic but without conflict. However, unhappiness and fighting can lead to stress.

Oftentimes, it's easy for parents to make adjustments in their schedules based on what someone else wants for them, such as a boss. It should be just as easy to do with a child's needs. It's a matter of priorities. Parents need to be willing to make changes and to be honest with themselves about how much attention they are really paying to their children. It's possible to rebalance your life without a

lot of work. The result is likely to be a happier child and a better relationship with that child.

If a child is unhappy about going to school, he or she may be
having problems in school, and may not want to admit it. Parents
need to be detectives, in a way. Try to speak to people at school to
find out what's happening. Look for subtle cues, such as a change in
behavior, sleep, or appetite, or more nervousness or preoccupations.
A change in schoolwork habits might clue you in to a potential
problem. Think about whether your child is in some new situation
that might lead to potential stress, and consider that your child may
be denying the stress (not consciously—they truly are "unaware" that
they are stressed). Note whether the change in behavior has occurred
about the same time as the potential source of stress. And be ready
to discuss things in general, and the stressful situation in particular, if
your child does decide to open up. Children are often upset when
they have to miss school, because they'll miss seeing their friends,
after-school activities, and they will have to make up work. When they
start having physical complaints and seem indifferent to missing
school (and are not "truly" sick), look for something about going to
school that is stressful, that the child may be avoiding.

Action Points

1. Look at how much time you spend with your children.
2. Rebalance your life so you can pay more attention to them.
3. Be a detective about school—ask specific questions about what's
   going on, but don't be too pushy, and follow your child's cues
   when they respond.
4. Be ready to discuss specific complaints, and to relate them to
   stressful situations

CHAPTER 11

How Your Child Relates to Family, Friends, and Role Models

*J*ames, age twelve, was having some problems with his soccer coach, and lately the tension had overflowed into his home and school life. He was trying out for the travel team, and was practicing three afternoons a week plus practicing or playing in games on the weekend. His coach tended to bark at the team, and benched players who did not play well.

"My mind is stuck thinking about playing and on the coach, who gets on me when I make a bad pass or bad shot. What does he expect? I know if I mess up, I won't play," says James. He kept much of this from his parents, fearing he'd disappoint them, though he became moody on soccer days.

One day after what seemed like a routine scuffle, James complained of knee pain. While he seemed to walk normally when he thought no one was looking, he limped when his parents came in the room, and told them he couldn't practice. After much prodding, his parents finally found out what was happening with the soccer coach. When confronted, the coach unfortunately was more interested in winning than in James's feelings. James decided that he could not play for this coach. He joined a more low-key league, and his knee pain, as well as his moodiness, soon vanished.

Translation: "That coach is a real 'pain in my knee,' and it's affecting me on and off the field."

A growing body of research suggests that a child's relationships are integral to self-esteem, mood, and overall development. These interpersonal relationships start with parents, but continue throughout childhood to include friends and role models. Clearly, how a child relates to others is important. Stable interpersonal relationships can help diminish the impact of conduct disorders. One study of teen depression done by Laura Mufson shows that interpersonal psychotherapy, which focuses on relationships, is quite effective. This chapter suggests that helping your child foster good person-to-person relationships might protect against depression and help a child develop socially. If a child is having problems interacting with other people, it's important to assess them early on.

Sibling Rivalry and Pressure to Perform

Our society puts a lot of pressure on younger siblings to perform. A younger child expects, and wants, to do as well as an older brother or sister. Family, friends, and teachers may implicitly or explicitly compare younger children to older siblings, sometimes unfairly. A younger sibling may not be as proficient, or may be behaviorally or physically challenged, which can lead to behavioral symptoms.

Siblings almost certainly do activities and play together, and much of the time they make up games that have winners or losers. Even in non-competitive activities—kicking a ball, swimming, bicycling—it's often evident when one child is better than another, and they are almost sure to point this out to each other.

Given my children's differences in both skills and interests, I've found it best to encourage them to try different things so that they don't compete directly with each other. My daughter Hannah has some different interests than her older sister Carly. Hannah likes and is good at tennis, and takes lessons regularly, but Carly doesn't. Carly, on the other hand, loves skateboarding, and goes to skateboarding camp. As your children get older, they shouldn't just be clones of one another. Every child has his or her own talents and interests. Part of your job as a parent is to identify and cultivate them.

I tell my children the goal of sports is to do their best and have fun, rather than winning, and point out that they can often learn more about what they need to do to develop skills further from losing than winning;

in this way, losing is viewed positively. But don't delude yourself that life is not competitive. It's a question of balance. You don't want to avoid competition, and, in fact, you want to find ways for your children to compete. By competing, they learn how to deal with winning and losing and are not at the mercy of their feelings if they don't win. But you don't want them constantly competing with each other.

When my children do compete, I try to emphasize it's just a game. To the winner, I'll say that on any given day, you may not win. To the loser, I'll praise the effort and say there's always another day. My main message is that if you're a winner and gloat, or if you're a sore loser, others won't like to play with you. And if my kids are being particularly vicious, I simply stop the game. I tell them that trying your hardest means that you are always a winner, no matter what the outcome.

When one sibling is physically or emotionally challenged, parents need to enlist the other siblings as allies to ensure they are protective and less competitive. Such preparation will help diminish the intensity of the inevitable competitive situations when they come up. Parents will focus on developing the differential abilities of the challenged child and strengthening his or her weaknesses.

Authority Figures

As children age, other adults become important in their lives and serve as surrogates for parents. Growing children spend more and more time outside the home, and are judged, taught, and critiqued by others. Depending upon how sensitive, skilled, and understanding these other adults are in their interactions with children, they have the potential to cause a traumatic experience for a child. When children have conflicts with these authority figures, they can do little about it. Parents need to be able to talk to their children and help them make connections between what's going on outside the home and how they feel. Teachers and other parents can help provide the feedback you may need.

Social Acceptance

Social acceptance is an important factor for developing self-esteem. Children begin to share ideas and feelings at an early age. They acquire social skills—how to share, listen, and be empathic—when they are included in groups as they grow up. They also assimilate social norms—many boys tend to cluster into group activities, often centered around sports, and play video and computer games, while girls tend to do more one-on-one activities such as talking and playing with each other (though more girls play team sports now). Girls, however, engage in more traditionally "male" gender activities and interests than the other way around, which has been quite positive for female development. If your eight-year-old boy has no idea what the "hottest" new game is that all the other boys are talking about and playing, or your fifteen-year-old girl still plays with dolls, they may have difficulty interacting with age mates socially. Observe how your child plays, and talk to other parents about how the child gets along with friends. Meet with your child's teacher and ask about how your child plays in organized activities.

Mirror, Mirror

From an early age, children mirror their self-image from their parents. Children need their parents' support, feedback, and involvement in what they're doing. Parents who are overly critical and put too much pressure on their children can affect self-esteem and the motivation to succeed negatively. If children are not motivated, they often have low energy and feel sad. Observing positive energy and positive coping skills in their parents helps them develop their own positive coping skills. Also, hopeful, confident parents do better emotionally than hopeless, pessimistic parents.

Sports and Development

Sports play a critical, often defining, role in the lives of children. Virtually all children have some experience with organized sports. But for many children, athletics in America has become an obsession, in both the negative and positive sense of the word. At times, the players are viewed only as athletes and not as children who happen to be playing sports.

It seems that spontaneous pickup games in neighborhoods and on school playgrounds are rapidly becoming a thing of the past. Structured, organized sports activities, run by adults, now dominate youth sports. This makes it imperative that parents become involved and develop a greater awareness of their children's developmental sports needs.

A developmental perspective is useful in understanding the changing abilities and needs of growing children, particularly when it comes to competitive sports. Parents who recognize the different developmental level can help children through changes in athletic abilities and interests.

Preschoolers and early grade school children may lack the physical, emotional, and cognitive (thinking) maturity to play many sports. What I mean is that they may not be physically capable of mastering the necessary skills, emotionally mature enough for competition, or able to understand and follow the rules. At these young ages, it's critical to give children positive feedback for their efforts, regardless of whether they win or lose. Negative feedback by parents, teachers, and coaches who dwell on the outcomes of games can have a devastating effect on a young child's self-esteem.

Many children drop out of organized youth sports between ages eight and thirteen, largely due to the poor quality of adult supervision and coaching and the amount of pressure parents place on young athletes to perform. On the other hand, a supportive sports environment can improve morale, performance, and physical competence. Boys and girls of this age say the things that motivate them to be involved in sports include improving skills, having fun, learning new skills, being challenged, and being physically fit, says Medical College of Pennsylvania psychiatrist Ronald Kamm, M.D. He believes the goal should be to encourage these behaviors through positive reinforcement and to instill action toward achievement rather than a fear of failure.

Teens typically crave greater independence, control, and autonomy. However, the emphasis on winning in structured, competitive sports may place stressful demands on adolescent athletes. Parents and coaches need to nurture, support, and encourage these athletes in a consistent way, and remember to respect the teen as a person as well as a player.

Today's teens often juggle social and academic activities along with extracurricular sports. Maintaining a balance is crucial to developing a strong personality. Too much isolated training, for example, a champion ice skater who works with a professional coach several hours a day, may disrupt normal social interactions and development.

Benefits of Sports

Through sports, children develop leadership, cooperativeness, team-work, self-discipline, and skills to help them deal with both adversity and success. They also learn respect for authority, competitiveness, sports-manship, and self-confidence. Youth sports can provide a healthy outlet for energy and expression. Sports can also help encourage social competence, family bonding, and facilitate friendships.

Participation in sports can have a therapeutic effect on a child's often fragile sense of self-esteem and belonging. Encouraging sports participation can help children optimize their capabilities. Associations have been made between sports participation and decreased teen pregnancy, higher academic achievement, including higher graduation rates from high school and college, decreased delinquency and recreational substance abuse, and higher self-esteem and lower depression rates, though more research is needed to prove these associations.

Many researchers have found that participating in aerobic exercise may also increase creativity, according to Florida State University educational researcher Lisa R. Herman-Tofler. So, children may make gains in the classroom as well as the ball fields as they exercise more.

Besides the physical benefits, moderate involvement in sports has been related to lower levels of depression among adolescents and a more positive outlook on life. In fact, young athletes with high self-esteem seem to cope better with general life stress. According to a study at the University of Western Australia in Perth led by I.W. Ford, the more self-assured and optimistic among the 121 athletes who competed in a variety of sports dealt with life changes better than those with lower self-esteem. And what's more, those with high self-esteem were less vulnerable to injuries and recovered faster from injuries.

Sports, Chronic Illness, and Disabilities

For a child with a chronic illness, sports participation may lead to a better self-image, less anxiety, and improved coping skills. Every illness seems to have its own successful role model—for example, Olympic gold medal swimmer Amy Van Dykens with asthma and former professional baseball player Jim Eisenreich with Tourette's syndrome.

Children with ADHD, learning disorders, and mood disorders may also benefit from playing sports by developing social skills and improving relationships with their peers. For children with impaired social skills or coordination problems, individual sports such as martial arts may provide a structure and sense of accomplishment, two critical factors in the development of physical well-being, self-esteem, and psychological growth.

Sports can have meaningful effects on children with developmental disabilities by helping to improve their physical and psychological functioning. Just look at the children who participate in the Special Olympics, the largest recreational sports program in the world for people with developmental disabilities. As you would expect, Special Olympians show improved physical fitness because they go through rigorous training. But they also have better self-esteem and show improved abilities to make friends and interact with their peers.

Sports Risks

Besides the physical risks of playing sports, children may be subject to emotionally stressful situations. Repeated failures, criticism, negative interactions with peers as well as overly ambitious pressures to perform may affect a child's psychological development and self-esteem. Inappropriate expectations of parents, coaches, and teammates can prevent even a good athlete from reaching his or her potential.

Excessive stress, anxiety, and pressure imposed by coaches, parents, and athletes themselves may lead to less-than-optimal performances and injuries that limit sports participation. Children subjected to these forces may be susceptible to moodiness, depression, chronic fatigue, substance abuse, and eating disorders. Young athletes wanting to avoid the stress of competition or intense participation may resort to malingering or even injure themselves on purpose. Stress may manifest itself as pain, injury, or weakness, with or without any physiological cause. For the young athlete, pain and injury can be an acceptable way to quit, decrease expectations, or escape high-pressured competition, without losing pride.

Coaches' Behavior

There is a relationship between coaching behaviors and sports anxiety in young athletes. For the majority of young people involved in sports, the coach is a strong influence. A coach's behavior toward physical training, mental preparation, goal setting, technical skills, and competition can affect a child's athletic performance, both positively and negatively.

Coaches who have a bad rapport with their youthful charges can induce anxiety. An Australian study led by J. Baker at the University of Queensland of 228 young athletes from various sports had the athletes complete a sports anxiety scale and a coaching behavior scale. The results show that a negative rapport between coach and athlete is an important contributor to an athlete's anxiety. In addition, coaches who had a good attitude about competition could lower an athlete's anxiety, reducing worries about winning and improving concentration.

Performance Enhancers

A "win at all costs" mentality is becoming increasingly common in youth sports, and coaches and young athletes often are looking for ways to improve performance and avoid sports injuries. The search for the "magic bullet" to improve performance has led some coaches to suggest young athletes try nutritional supplements. Various vitamins and herbal mixtures sold through catalogs advertised in muscle magazines purportedly improve strength. The variety of performance-enhancing drugs includes caffeine, amphetamines, human growth hormone, erythropoietin, thyroid hormone, human chorionic gonadotropin, gamma hydroxy butyrate, chromium picolinate, and anabolic steroids. Products known as ergogenic aids, designed to chemically improve sports performance, are quite popular among adolescent athletes. These and other nutritional supplements are billed as "natural" and "safe." But none of these products has been tested in or approved for use in young children or adolescents.

Aggressive coaches may also suggest strength training using anabolic steroids to improve muscle strength. The medical issues surrounding the use of these insidious drugs don't seem to bother coaches who just want results. From 4 to 12 percent of teenage boys and up to 2 percent of teenage girls may use anabolic steroids, according to a review of the field led by University of Michigan psychiatrist Kirk Brower, M.D. Boys involved in strength-related sports, such as football, wrestling, and bodybuilding, are the most likely group to use anabolic steroids. This group of steroid users is also more likely to use illicit drugs, alcohol, and tobacco.

Very few side effects of steroid use are immediately apparent, so young athletes may continue using steroids and ignore the serious medical implications. The excess of male hormones circulating in the blood can cause a personality change toward increased aggressiveness and irritability, mood swings, and even psychotic episodes. Serious side effects of steroid use include impotence, sterility, kidney, liver, and heart function changes, and an increased risk of liver cancer.

Action Plan

First, assess how your child is relating to important people in his or her life. How does your child relate to siblings, peers, and others? Does your child get invited to get-togethers or parties? Do friends call or e-mail? Do friends come over when they are invited? Does your child have different sources of friendships through school, clubs, or a religious institution, or is your child overly dependent on one or two friends? Also look at how your child gets along with coaches and teachers. Does your child enjoy going to practice, lessons, or clubs?

Children compare themselves to each other all of the time in every way. They compare how many friends they have, how good they are at sports or at schoolwork, and how they look, talk, and dress. Whether you like it or not, they play computer games or one-on-one basketball together, where there's always a winner and a loser. Each child has different talents or challenges that affect the outcomes of competition. Since comparing is an everyday circumstance, I try to minimize the amount my children compete. Instead, what's important is learning how to interact, and how to try one's best. If children learn that at home, they can take it into interactions with their friends.

Sometimes, as parents, we compare one child to another, either implicitly or explicitly. You may look at all of your children's report cards together and unwittingly begin to compare how many check marks or high numbers each child has. In our house, my wife and I avoid that by opening up, and going over, each child's report card separately. It's hard sometimes because they want to see each others' report cards. So whether you do it or not, be aware of comparing children. Know that they compare themselves with their siblings, and try not to feed into it.

To help reduce siblings' comparisons, encourage them to pursue different activities, as well as sharing in some of the same activities. Maybe they can be on separate teams or play different musical instruments. Sometimes children won't agree—they may insist on doing what their big sister did. If they do, then try hard to avoid explicitly comparing them, such as, saying to one, "Why can't you be as organized as your brother?"

When it comes to after-school activities, such as sports, parents need to be parents. By that, I mean go to practices and games and really watch. Observe how much your child relates to teammates and the coach. Don't just be there. Pay attention to your child on and off the field. Sometimes parents overdo it, which has led some communities to set policies that don't allow parents to abuse coaches on the field. I say or do little more than encourage my children during games. If you really feel you need to confront a coach, do it before or after a practice or game or by phone when your children are out of earshot.

If you see that your child is upset about something, talk about it on the way home or later on. For example, you might say, "I noticed that when Coach took you out, you were angry." Or "When you missed that shot, I saw you looked upset." Give your child a chance to express his or her feelings, and provide an empathetic shoulder to cry on, if necessary. A little encouragement, particularly for a younger child, goes a long way.

Regardless of the role of adults involved with your children—a coach, group leader, or camp counselor—schedule the equivalent of a teacher conference every so often. Besides school, some places have built-in mechanisms for regular interactions, for example, visiting day the middle weekend of a two-week overnight camp. Too often, parents fail to get feedback on how their child is doing. If nothing formal is set up, do it yourself. Parents don't usually sit in on music lessons, but you can ask for a regular update on how your child is performing, whether it's above or below everyone's expectations. Again, one or the other parent should regularly attend activities, games, or recitals as much as possible.

With regular feedback, you can troubleshoot along the way. If your child is not happy after practice, discuss it with your child and the coach to avoid turning it into a bigger problem than it is. Just as you might speak to your child's teacher about getting extra help in a subject before the child flunks that first test, speak to your child's coach or music teacher about what areas your child needs to work on to help enhance performance and self-esteem.

You can do the same investigative work when it comes to friendships. If your child seems not be invited to places by others or invites no friends to your home, start by getting information from the child's teacher. School is the main source of friendships for most children. If the teacher says your child often goes off by himself, but others are accepting or solicitous of him, try to elicit more information from him. Is he nervous, or depressed? If your child is annoying others, find out whether she is aware that she does that. Often, the teacher can facilitate interactions with classmates. Interventions may range from you or the teacher talking to the child to a further evaluation if you think significant anxiety, depression, or a behavioral problem may be interfering with your child's functioning.

One way to help a child's interaction with friends is to arrange or structure play dates. Once children enter elementary school, they may want to arrange their own play dates or ask for help in setting them up. For younger children, parents generally have to arrange play dates for their children. When the children are together, watch how they relate to each other and to see whether it's going well. Check out whether your child shares well, tends to ignore the other child, or does not play nicely, for example, is not a good loser or a gracious winner.

Parents should try to develop an early sense of the child's social style. Talk about what goes on in school and during play dates to get a sense of how your child acts and reacts to various situations. This knowledge will help you find out what works best when you need to correct a younger child during a play date. For an older child, if you notice a problem in progress, ask to speak to the child separately for a second.

For children with lots of social problems who do poorly engaging another child in an activity, a parent can suggest something to do. If a child has social problems in reading other children or responding to social cues (such as picking up on it when a friend is lukewarm toward doing a specific activity, or is wandering off to do something by herself), invite them to do a fun thing together, such as going to a park, a baseball game, a movie, or out to dinner. Parents do that with their friends. This is not bribing. I see it as a suggestion that might well help cement a friendship and give parents a way to stay close by and have an idea of what's going on during the play date.

Children notice how parents interact with their own friends. Be conscious that you are always on stage for your children, and that they will react to what they see. If your child watches you play a competitive game, he or she will notice how much you are affected by it. If you lose, try to work through it and let it go. You don't need to present unrealistic models to follow. If you're frustrated about losing, that's part of life. It's how you deal with the frustration that's more important.

When you play games with your children, you need to walk a fine line. If you always let your child win, neither of you have fun, and your child may be humiliated because you are not trying your best. But beating your child all of the time isn't fun either. Try to approximate how a child that age would play so you can make it fun for both of you. Take pleasure in the fact that your child is developing skills, and is not afraid to use them.

It is important for children to enjoy themselves during preschool as they learn and master fundamental sports skills. This enables them to feel competent as they play a variety of sports during elementary school. As parents, we need to provide support and encouragement as we teach growing youngsters to play sports, and to foster this sense of competence. Teens need to have the opportunity to develop a sense of mastery on their own, to manage themselves emotionally, and to learn to cope with adversity.

Playing sports at all levels can be fun and rewarding. Parents must not lose sight of their children's needs to develop the self-esteem that enables them to face the challenges of adulthood. Competition and stress are integral to modern life. But stressful competition should never overwhelm the primary goals of playing sports—having fun, building appropriate developmental skills, both physical and emotional, and enhancing relationships with peers.

Not all children with developmental disabilities are inclined to join a basketball or swimming team, but they all can benefit from an appropriate exercise program. As parents, your job is to help them realize the many benefits of sports and exercise.

Parents sometimes recognize their athletic child only for his sports achievements. These parents need to clarify their priorities. Athletic success should not be placed above a child's psychological and physical health. Here are some questions from University of California at Los Angeles psychiatrist Barri Stryer, M.D., to ask yourself, as a parent of a child athlete, to help you get a handle on how you perceive your child's involvement in sports:

- Do you consider your child underinvolved, moderately involved, or overinvolved in sports?
- What are your child's and your family's level of involvement in sports? Do you attend your child's games as a spectator, a coach, or a referee?
- How do you model behavior for your child (for example, when your child's team loses)?
- How do family members (mother, father, siblings, and grandparents) participate in sports: as nonathletes, interested spectators, enthusiastic amateurs, aspiring elitists, professional athletes, or coaches?
- What do you do for fun and relaxation?

Children long for their parents' approval, and readily identify with their attitudes and values, both good and bad. How parents and coaches act is an excellent predictor of how a child will behave while playing sports since they are their main role models. Children of physically active parents are more likely to participate in sports, and they also receive greater encouragement to participate when their parents enjoy their own involvement in sports. Coaches exert an increasing influence on the sports interest and participation of older children and teens, but parents can still play supportive roles.

University of Pittsburgh psychiatrist Stuart Libman, M.D., has devised parenting tasks for youth sports as a child ages. For preschoolers, he suggests that parents introduce the child to a variety of sports, emphasize fun and skill development, and offer encouragement and positive feedback. For those in elementary school, parents should provide opportunities to rehearse sports skills; create an atmosphere of interest, support, and playfulness; and promote involvement in the sports preferred by the child. During adolescence, the parent's job is to support participation in preferred sports activities; relinquish coaching responsibilities, if possible; and continue to monitor overall development.

Coaching offers the opportunity not only to teach children a particular sport, but also to influence them to expand their identity, develop self-esteem, and increase their capacity to cope with life's demands. Competitive team sports can also teach values about cooperation and teamwork, and coaches can present competition as a way to challenge the child by striving to perform at the highest level.

Yet, most recreational sports coaches in communities have no formal training, and the training of school coaches varies widely. Typically, coaches have little knowledge of physiologic or psychological development and the healthiest ways to instruct children. They may not possess the ability to tactfully communicate with young athletes and their parents. Coaches need to remember that each child develops physically and mentally at different rates. A child who might appear to have less athletic potential might simply be developing abilities at a different pace. I recommend that any parent considering coaching take a Coach Effectiveness Training course, a well-researched program for training youth sport coaches.

Dr. Libman has also outlined coaching tasks for youth sports as a child ages. At the preschool level, coaches may teach fundamental sports skills, and provide fun, cooperative, noncompetitive sports activities and games. For elementary-age children, the coach provides repetitive instruction and emotional support, and promotes mastery of physical and mental skills in specific sports. For adolescents, the coach provides advanced instruction in skills and knowledge, and fosters internal performance standards and promotes mental toughness.

To enhance their performance, teen athletes can learn stress-reduction skills. Techniques such as deep breathing, relaxation, and imagery, together with skills to mentally correct for errors, can enable a young athlete to become more confident in managing the stress of competition. Players can be taught to use their mental skills to review past athletic events and to prepare for upcoming contests. Their capacity for resilience in the face of adversity is a way to promote mental toughness.

Mental toughness is not just about enhancing athletic performance but about dealing effectively with life's challenges. These mental skills not only enhance athletic performance but teach valuable coping skills that translate to success off the field.

A strength-training program that's properly designed and supervised—without performance enhancers—is a great idea. Influencing adolescent athletes' attitudes toward steroids requires more than merely presenting information about the medical consequences of their use. Providing alternatives to performance-enhancing drugs, such as advice about good nutrition and weightlifting techniques, may be more effective in discouraging steroid use. Enhancing your child's self-esteem may also help prevent steroid use.

Possible indicators of steroid use include rapid increases in muscle size or strength, obsessive focus with weightlifting and diet, preoccupation with body image, increased appetite, and mood swings. If you suspect your child is using anabolic steroids, a trip to the doctor and laboratory tests can provide useful feedback about their possible harmful effects. These tests should include liver function tests, a cholesterol profile, hormone tests, and a complete blood workup. A semen analysis may also reveal decreased sperm count.

Most of the complications of steroid use are reversible by stopping the drugs. During this initial period off steroids, parents should watch for suicidal thoughts. Antidepressants may be prescribed if your child becomes depressed. Some children may need hospitalization, but reassurance, education, and counseling are the recommended treatments during withdrawal from steroids.

Many anabolic steroid users rely on their physical appearance to maintain their self-esteem. Others may continue to feel physically small no matter how big they get while using steroids. Psychotherapy may help children develop a balance of sports and other pursuits that can lead to feelings of competence.

Action Points

1. Assess how your child relates to the people in his or her life.
2. Recognize that children compare themselves to each other all of the time—so do you. Try not to encourage it.
3. Watch your child compete, and help him or her deal with the feelings of winning and losing.
4. Ask your child's teacher, coach, or instructor for specific feedback on what areas may need more effort or work, and be involved in programs that promote the training of coaches to help them understand how to best deal with children.
5. Be involved with your children's friendships. Watch how they play.
6. Watch how you respond to winning or losing; your child is watching your reactions.
7. Support and encourage young athletes to make sports fun.
8. Become a physically active role model.
9. Enhance your child's self-esteem to help prevent steroid use, and get help from your pediatrician if you suspect that your child is using steroids.

CHAPTER 12

Not Absolutely Perfect—
How to Cope with Normal Childhood

Six-year-old Liam couldn't wait for his summer vacation at the beach with his family. For weeks, he strutted around the house, brimming with excitement. Nearly every day he asked, "Mom, how many more days?" When he finally arrived at the beach, however, Liam did an abrupt about-face. "I don't like this place. I can't sleep in that bed, and I miss Cocoa (the family dog). I want to go home!" he shrieked. Later, at a restaurant, he yelled, "I don't like this food," which he had picked from the children's menu. Liam's mom, Pat, felt her blood pressure rising. "I couldn't believe it," Pat said. "I thought this was going to be the most wonderful time. Then he just snapped. He really fooled me."

Translation: "Going on vacation overwhelms me. I'm tired from the long car ride, which makes me moody. I don't like being in an unfamiliar place, sleeping in a strange bed, and eating different food."

Most parents take great pains to ease their children through major traumas such as divorce or moving to a new neighborhood, but they often overlook the other things that children find stressful. Normal day-to-day situations trigger the most common stress for children. Enjoyable events, such as a birthday party, family gatherings, or a vacation can quickly overload a child's circuits. Even seemingly minor concerns—such as a fear of the dark or being teased by a bully—can snowball into serious anxiety for a child whose parents don't help put things into perspective.

Lazy, Hazy, Crazy Days of Childhood

While children are often not concerned about very much, it's misleading to think that children have no concerns. Children do worry and have fears. How much they worry depends on their developmental level, temperament, life experience, coping models, and other environmental factors.

Parents may assume that children react the same way as adults do to stress. But stress affects children differently. Developmentally, they may lack the cognitive ability to really understand stressful events.

I encourage parents to have children talk about themselves, their activities, and most importantly, their feelings. Talking together is a perfect opportunity to enhance a child's self-esteem and to help the child overcome the feeling of helplessness that often accompanies everyday anxieties and stress.

Where Does Stress Come From?

Stress comes from everywhere. The real issue is whether the amounts of stress a child experiences overtax his or her capabilities or reserves. Extreme stress or chronic, unremitting stress during sensitive periods of development can affect a child's emotional and physical health.

A child's age seems to be the greatest predictor of how a child responds to stress. Adolescent angst about looks and popularity are well recognized, but preschoolers' stresses are more subtle. Among children ages three to five, common stressors include going to school for the first time, conflicts with siblings, having to temper emerging independence with increasing demands from their parents (toilet training, cleaning up after themselves, etc.), family vacations away from home, and unfamiliar experiences, such as having a new sitter or playing at a friend's house where Mom or Dad are not close at hand.

For children between ages six and ten, the most stressful situations generally relate to school—beginning a new school year, keeping up with academics and taking tests, being chosen for teams, and trying to please teachers. Other stressful situations include making friends and being accepted socially and pleasing authority figures other than teachers, including parents. Children can be very sensitive to subtle social nuances. A shove on the playground or a giggle on the bus can be serious stuff for children.

Significant illnesses or an illness in the family, family moves, a school or teacher change can also lead to major stress. For more complete information on the stresses of childhood, see Chapter 14.

Exciting Events

Exciting events may cause hidden stress. A child might feel stress about her birthday party not because she is excited, but because she is uncomfortable being the center of attention when "Happy Birthday" is sung. Or maybe the child does not have the social skills to manage all of her friends at once. Getting a new pet can be exciting, yet may stir up fears of not knowing how to care for the pet or worries that a young pet has been separated from its parent.

Too Much Stimulation

Too many activities can lead to stress overload. Piling on after-school music lessons and sports, plus homework, may get to be too much. Parents need to help their children set priorities so that a workable, manageable schedule can be arranged to provide plenty of unstructured time for relaxation. They can also help children plan ahead for upcoming stressful events, such as a recital or a big game.

Stress can motivate children to get things done, solve problems, or take on challenges. It's a question of the type and intensity of stress as well as the child's disposition and stress-coping skills.

Put Things in Perspective

Because children may not have yet developed their reasoning skills, little things can easily get blown out of proportion. A first grader may see only a scary monster lurking in strange shadows. In the same way, it often doesn't occur to older children that a friend who doesn't return a phone call may just be busy or that a sibling who snaps at them may have had a bad day.

Children are often victims of their own misinterpretations. Very plainly, parents need to put things into perspective for them. I encourage parents to listen sympathetically without making judgments or brushing off children's concerns, which can make matters worse. When you take their little problems seriously, children will feel respected and that they can trust you and will likely confide in you when something deeply troubles them.

Some of the signs that children are on the negative side of the seesaw of stress management include: sleep and appetite problems, irritability, defiant behavior, or recurrent illnesses. The ultimate research linking the social stress of deprivation in foundling homes to infectious illness and death was Rene Spitz's research on orphaned children raised in foundling hospitals in the mid-twentieth century. He found that one-third of infants in foundling homes died by one year of age. This dramatic example underscores the connection between the stress of social deprivation and susceptibility to physical illness.

Action Plan

The first step is to analyze your child's behavior rather than just react to it. Your feelings may interfere with your perception of what's really affecting your child. A parent can easily get lost in feeling unappreciated. Remember, children often react to stress without being consciously aware of the situation. Your job is to figure out what may have caused the stress and help your child make a transition away from the stress.

Sometimes, that's easier said than done. Take a step back, and put aside your own expectations, because your expectations of your child and what he or she can handle might not be realistic. You can't force a child to mold to your expectations. Yes, it can be frustrating, but parents need to learn how to manage the disparity between their child's behavior and their own expectations.

Stress affects each child differently. What might stress one child might not stress another. So you can't look at an event and decide whether it should or should not affect your child. Stress does what it does. And your child has a right to be stressed.

You can't avoid all stressful situations for your child. They are going to happen, no matter what. It's best not to deny or ignore the stress. Think of stress as environmentally shaping your child's strengths. Also, try not to invalidate the stress because of your own expectations. Don't ask, "Why are you stressed out?" in a way that implies the child should not be stressed. That question projects your own opinion about what should be stressful. Instead, help your child through the stress to get to a positive outcome.

If you really can't decipher your child's behavior, look at the domains outlined earlier in this book for clues to ongoing and acute stresses. Ongoing stress may occur when your child struggles with math or a bully at school for the whole year; or a parent is ill for several months or has a chronic disability. Acute stress may be precipitated by a failing grade, a fight in school, or a parent admitted to the hospital.

Don't be fooled by whether you consider the stressful event to be happy or sad. Rather than ascribing a positive or negative feeling to the event, think about it as a process. What might be happy for one child may be sad for another. For example, if one child does well on a test, but her twin fails the same test, it may be a bittersweet moment.

There's a fine line between helping a child through a situation with some coping skills and realizing it's best to back off and not push the issue. Your reaction depends on how important the event or issue is in the overall context of your child's life.

When it comes to tantrums, safety is the first priority. If your child is going to hurt himself or someone else, you have to take steps to prevent any harm. Try to understand why the child is upset. You might state your understanding of the situation to the child, but it is unlikely that the child will be able to listen during the tantrum. Instead, use that understanding to guide your intervention in the situation, without labeling.

Try not to get lost in the tantrum. Your child may kick a waste can or call you an idiot. Instead of adding on punishments for each infraction, try to defuse the situation. Most times, the best initial reaction is to ignore the child. You can't bang your head against the wall if someone removes the wall. Also, you may just be giving your child negative attention by focusing on the tantrum. After your child calms down, investigate what might have caused the problem.

Parents are spin doctors. You can make stressful things seem positive. Think of it as a challenge. You'll feel good, or less pained, when you're successful and your child calms down.

In the end, step back and check your own expectations. Treat your child as an individual regardless of whether you think it's reasonable. Come up with a constructive outcome in a positive way. Don't purely react to your child's behavior itself. For routine tantrums caused by acute stress, try to ride them out. Put a positive spin on the situation using distraction or enticements. If the situation gets to the point where your child is having significant, recurrent tantrums on a daily basis and you can't get them under control, then it may be time for input from your pediatrician and a mental health professional. For a look at potential psychiatric problems, see the sections on anxiety and depression in Chapter 7.

Action Points

1. Analyze, don't just react to, your child's behavior. Try to figure out what might be the cause of stress.
2. Help your child through the stress to a positive outcome.
3. Be a spin doctor—put a positive spin on the situation using distraction or enticements. This is no more "fake" than calling the glass "half full" instead of "half empty." Even when a child struggles or has a setback, focus on what positive can come from it.
4. Ride out tantrums by first ignoring them and then investigating the cause. If they happen often, seek help from a professional.

CHAPTER 13

How Are You Doing, Mom and Dad—
Stress Rolls Downhill

One of my patients, Devin, a nine-year-old boy, was having difficulties with his mood, and how he was getting along with other kids. He had mood swings and was not able to let go of things. His mother, Mary, told me she felt overwhelmed and hopeless, and was very negative about him. Mary's outlook was starting to affect her interactions with Devin. His father, Jeff, was relatively uninvolved in Devin's life and was not helping out much raising this difficult child. After several efforts, Jeff finally agreed to come in with Devin and Mary to see me, and he agreed to set up monthly visits to discuss how he could be more involved in his son's life. Jeff liked athletic activities and was interested in watching sporting events, but Devin wasn't interested in either. Jeff had a hard time relating to his son. Through regular visits along with his wife, Jeff began to recognize the importance of finding a way to connect with his son and be an active presence in his life. They began to play board games together and to visit museums and other places Devin was interested in. Jeff also agreed to spend less time watching sports events on television. Spending more time with his son helped Mary and reduced her stress level. She was more able to deal with Devin's behavior, felt less angry with her husband, and the situation at home improved almost immediately.

Translation (Mom): "I'm stressed-out, and that's affecting my son. I wish my husband would help me out with our son, but he can't seem to relate to him."

As parents you don't have to look in the mirror to see whether you are under stress. Just look at your children. They'll tell you—with their actions more than words—whether you're stressed-out. This chapter describes how parents' stress and parenting styles can affect children, and reviews how stress affects parents and how they can reduce their own stress levels. I'm calling for parents to give their children time and affection and the kind of caring and sharing that allows children to grow up feeling good about themselves.

Children See, Children Do

Poor parenting skills may cause children undue stress. Constant nagging and threats slowly eat away at children's good feelings about themselves. Children who have poor role models may have inadequate or inappropriate coping skills for stress.

Mostly, children learn best from parents who demonstrate self-control by using effective stress-coping skills. The feelings and moods of family members do rub off on each other. This is called "reciprocity." Parents can establish a positive emotional chain reaction with their children by showing them how to cope well with stress.

Anger and Blood Pressure

A parent's anger can raise a child's blood pressure, even if the anger isn't aimed at the child. A study of thirty-four four- and five-year-olds reported in *Pediatrics for Parents* found that listening to tapes of adults arguing raised the children's blood pressure, which is a signal of stress. During the study, the children's mothers were present. The increase in blood pressure isn't significant itself, but shows how parents actions can adversely affect their children.

Stressed Moms, Stressed Babes

Research among primates shows that if moms are stressed, so are their babies. While it's a long leap from primates to humans, this information gives us another clue about how stressed parents can affect their children.

Research by Columbia University psychiatrist Jeremy Coplan, M.D., and colleagues looked at how monkeys respond to stress, and how their response affects their infants. Their evidence suggests that monkeys' adverse early experiences, such as not knowing when they would eat, can affect the future development of major psychiatric disorders among adults. corticotropin-releasing factor (CRF), a natural brain chemical, regulates the stress response in mammals. In one of Coplan's studies, adult monkeys that were exposed as infants to stressful conditions were studied to determine if long-term changes of CRF had occurred following this early stress. In comparison to monkeys reared by mothers looking for food under predictable conditions, infant monkeys raised by mothers foraging under unpredictable conditions had high concentrations of CRF that remained that way even after they grew up. High levels of CRF are believed to contribute to certain psychological disorders, including anxiety. This finding explains why stress early in life may contribute to psychological problems in adulthood. It is theorized that this biological system (CRF) may be linked to psychiatric disorders in humans.

If this primate data applies to humans, stress in pregnant mom's may affect the central nervous system development of their infants.

Other studies at Stanford University, among others, suggest that infant monkeys who are subjected to prolonged separations from their moms also have increased levels of cortisol. In one experiment at the National Institute of Alcohol Abuse and Alcoholism led by Claudia Fahlke, these same monkeys were more likely to drink alcohol as adults!

Mother and Child Communion

Early parenting difficulties have also been associated with the development of asthma among children who are genetically at risk for the disease, which is the most common chronic illness of childhood. Researchers from the Mayo Clinic and Colorado asthma specialists studied 150 children with a family history of asthma over eight years. The children were considered genetically at risk for asthma because all of their mothers and some of their fathers had asthma.

They found parenting difficulties assessed in the first three weeks of life were significantly and independently associated with asthma when the children reached school age. Children whose parents had caretaking

difficulties had double the risk of developing asthma. The parenting difficulties noted included mother's depressed mood and coping problems,
relationship conflicts between the parents, an absence of social support,
and problems in providing sensitive, responsive caregiving.

Asthma is a complex disease with many contributing factors. Many of
the children in the study with well-adjusted, caring, effective parents still
developed asthma. But the results do indicate that the psychological environment of the child may play a role in the development of asthma. Emotional distress experienced early in life can have long-term health
consequences. It's important not to blame parents, but to support them in
doing their best to provide a nurturing environment.

The study also corroborates previous reports that an elevated blood
level of the antibody immunoglobulin E is associated with later development of asthma is this at-risk group.

Other asthma studies have found that parents of asthmatic children
tend to feel their child is stressed from severe asthma, while the children
themselves don't feel that anxious about the disease. So severe asthma
may stress the parents more than their affected children.

The mothers of children with recurrent abdominal pain also may over-
rate the effects on their children's emotional health. Studies have shown
that these mothers report that their children have more physical symptoms
and depression than their children reported. The more the mothers were
distressed about the tummy problems, the greater the difference between
what they reported and what their child reported about the pain.

Family stress may lead children who have irritable bowel syndrome
(IBS) to complain more of symptoms and to miss more days of school.
A study at Group Health Cooperative, a large health maintenance organization in Seattle, led by Rona Levy from the University of Washington in
Seattle, found that family stress and behavioral problems are associated
with more gastrointestinal (GI) symptoms and school absences. The study
included 141 children of women with IBS and 178 children of women with
no IBS. Children's symptoms were assessed by the Child Symptom Checklist. The mothers were asked about school absences and doctor visits,
and completed the Child Behavior Checklist and rated family stress on
another inventory. The researchers found that stress significantly correlated with GI symptoms, and all symptoms, reported by the children.
Stress also correlated with the number of disability days for GI and other

illnesses. Similarly, the scores on the behavior checklist correlated with GI symptoms and disability days for all illnesses, more so for boys than for girls. The conclusion was that both family stress and the number of problem behaviors were significantly related to children's GI symptoms and to GI-related school absenteeism.

Interestingly, the same group of researchers, led by William White-head from the University of North Carolina, looked at why recurrent tummyaches may be more common in large families, and whether this might be due to family stress or to attention-seeking. They looked at the same group of children whose mothers did or did not have IBS. The mothers were asked how many days in the last three months a child had missed school for GI symptoms and respiratory symptoms. Each child's perception that physical symptoms were rewarded with increased attention was assessed, as was family stress, with rating scales. The researchers found that having more than one sibling was associated with more GI symptoms reported by the children, more cold symptoms, and more symptoms of all kinds. These differences were still significant after they had been adjusted statistically for family stress.

Family stress was significantly related to the number of GI symptoms and all symptoms. Children with two or more brothers and sisters perceived that their mothers paid more attention to their GI symptoms than children with fewer siblings. The conclusion: children with multiple siblings reported more GI symptoms and other symptoms, which appear to be associated with mothers paying more attention to the physical complaints of children in large families.

Why Zebras Don't Get Ulcers

Your mental state can affect your physical health. This concept has spawned a new science called "psychoneuroimmunology," which has documented that stress causes changes in the immune system. There is little doubt that stress can affect health. Doctors know that stress can precipitate an asthma attack, and has been associated with chronic fatigue, insomnia, some gastrointestinal symptoms, migraine and tension headaches, and chronic back pain. Stress triggers a number of biochemical changes in the body, and can affect heart function, hormone levels, the nervous system, and metabolic rates. Psychoneuroimmunologists have concluded that stress appears to be the common denominator of many illnesses ranging from the common cold to heart disease to cancer.

The book *Why Zebras Don't Get Ulcers* by Robert Sapolsky gives lots of examples of how prolonged stress causes or intensifies a range of physical and mental afflictions, including depression, ulcers, colitis, heart disease, and immune system disorders. New research continues to show that psychological stress appears to undermine the body's resistance to infection.

Stress may increase susceptibility to infectious disease, according to Ohio State researchers Ronald Glaser and his wife Janice Kiecolt-Glaser, who have spent years studying the effects of stress on the body's immune system. They now believe they know enough to show that stress actually does weaken a person's health. Dozens of studies have shown that stress can alter the levels of certain biochemical markers in the body, called "cytokines," which are key players in the human immune response. But researchers weren't sure those changes actually lead to poorer health.

Now, they seem convinced. The researchers argue that stress can lessen a person's immune response and make that person more suscep- tible to infectious diseases. They also say that increased stress may lessen the effectiveness of certain vaccines and can confound some studies of certain illnesses that affect the immune system, such as AIDS and autoimmune diseases. The evidence so far suggests that while the immune changes associated with psychological stress are generally small, they appear to be important enough to have biological consequences and increase health risks.

Spanish research shows a relationship between a person's level of psychological stress and susceptibility to catching the common cold. To investigate whether stress increased the likelihood of developing a cold, the researchers surveyed more than 1,100 Spanish university staff and stu- dents at regular intervals over a one-year period. The study homed in on different types of stress, including stressful life events, perceived stress, and having a generally negative outlook and neurotic personality com- pared with a positive and extroverted one. Individuals with a negative out- look were at greatest risk of developing colds regardless of their use of vitamin C and zinc, and their smoking and drinking habits. Those at next highest risk were individuals who believed that they were under stress.

These people were nearly three times as likely as those with a positive outlook to develop a cold, the researchers report.

Stressed-Out People May Be Depressed

People who tell their doctor they're feeling stressed-out and have a long list of health complaints may be suffering from depression, anxiety, or other emotional problems.

Researchers from the Uniformed Services University of the Health Sciences in Bethesda, Maryland, found that, based on a questionnaire, more than one-quarter of 250 adult clinic patients were experiencing depression, anxiety, or some other emotional problems. One in ten patients had at least two emotional problems.

What's more, those who had experienced recent stress were nearly seven times more likely to have an underlying mental disorder. Those with at least six physical complaints faced four times the usual risk of having emotional problems. Just the feeling of having less than very good overall health more than doubled the risk of having mental problems.

Because doctors often do not pick up on such emotional problems—which people may be reluctant to talk about, or may even be unaware of—many people do not get the help they truly need. Patients with physical complaints as a manifestation of depression or anxiety will have significant improvement in their physical symptoms when the emotional problem is recognized and treated appropriately.

Reduce Stress, Boost Immunity

On the positive side, training in relaxation, stress reduction, and coping strategies may not only aid women psychologically, but also help them fight off breast cancer, according to David Spiegel, M.D. from Stanford University. Women with metastatic breast cancer who participated in a group psychological intervention program showed lower levels of the stress hormone cortisol and higher levels of an antibody that fights breast tumors than did other patients. In addition, women in the program were more likely than others to get the full dosage of their chemotherapy, showed lower levels of depression, and reported higher quality of life.

The encouraging news is that psychological interventions have reliable biological effects that can benefit women with breast cancer. The results are the first experimental data to show a link between psychological interventions and an immune response directly related to fighting breast cancer.

Interestingly, the same thing was found with men who had malignant melanoma in research by University of California at Los Angeles psychiatrist F. Fawzy. He and his colleagues evaluated the recurrence and survival for sixty-eight patients with malignant melanoma in a randomized, controlled study. Half received structured psychiatric group intervention for six weeks shortly after their diagnosis and initial surgery five to six years earlier, and half had no psychiatric intervention. The researchers found those who had the group intervention showed a trend toward fewer recurrences and had a lower death rate than the control group.

Studies like these will help us firm up the suspicion that reducing stress can strengthen the body's immune response.

Hypnosis and the Immune System

The same Ohio State researchers led by the Glasers have also determined that hypnosis used as a relaxation technique can actually prevent the weakening of the immune response that often follows acute stress. The research, reported in the *Journal of Consulting and Clinical Psychology*, is the latest to test whether people can protect themselves from immune system changes that normally accompany increased stress.

Hypnosis is used as something like "hitting a reset button" to help people shut out distracting thoughts and allow them to focus on the task at hand. In this study, half of thirty-three medical and dental students facing tough, highly stressful exams were taught self-hypnosis as a relaxation technique, while the other half served as controls. Those who used self-hypnosis before taking the tests showed a marked improvement in measurements of certain white blood cells, T lymphocytes, which are important to the immune response.

The more frequently the students in the hypnosis group practiced their technique, the better their immune response was. Only those who continued to practice hypnosis continued to have enhanced immune systems. The findings suggest that hypnosis or other relaxation techniques are most useful when people practice them consistently.

The interaction between stress and disease is much more complicated than the simplistic statement that someone under stress is likely to get sick. If that were true, anytime someone in your office had a cold, you would have one, too. Each person's immune system fights infections differently.

Likewise, we each cope with life's stresses differently. Stress comes not only from the environment but also from how we react to it. We can all learn how to cope better with potentially stressful situations.

Coping with Stress

How can parents cope better with stress? First, follow your mother's advice—get adequate amounts of rest, eat right, exercise regularly, and stay in contact with family and friends. No one thing can help you reduce stress. Instead, learn a variety of stress-management techniques, and use the ones that work best for you.

Relaxation Techniques

Parents who feel they are about to explode at their children can learn to use relaxation techniques such as breathing exercises and progressive muscle relaxation to help dissipate their tension. Deep breathing can bring the fast, shallow breaths of stress back to normal. Progressive muscle relaxation involves tensing, then relaxing, muscles, starting from the toes and working up the body to the neck and facial muscles.

The easiest and most common method of clearing the mind is through breathing, either by concentrating on the breath or breathing in conjunction with a focus word, says Columbia's Candace Erickson, M.D. The focus can also be a phrase, short prayer, or an image that helps to quiet the mind's chatter. Keep the focus word or phrase short, such as "relax," "calm," "peace," or "let go."

Using a focus word, breathe in, mentally counting from one to four, then breathe out, counting down from four to one. Count ten slow, deep breaths. Breathe out deeply, consciously letting go of your stress, then breathe in imagining that you are filling yourself with peace.

You can also combine awareness of breath with a physical focus. Massage your forehead, jaw, back of the neck, and shoulders. Stretch and yawn. Take a short walk, counting four paces as you breath in and four paces as you breathe out. Coordinate your breath with any activity, for example, jogging, lifting weights, vacuuming, or washing dishes.

You might also choose an image to focus on—a place you've been to, a scene in a picture, or a place you've imagined. Picture yourself in a relaxing place. Think of a picture of a nature scene. Imagine what it would feel like to be a tree (strong, rooted), a mountain (timeless, stable), a wave (fluid, limitless), the sun (radiant, warm), or the wind (free, floating).

Practice these techniques when you're not under stress once or twice a day. There's also a self-hypnosis technique in Chapter 15. Find the ones that suit you best, or invent your own ways to take a minibreak.

Quiet, Quality Time

Parents may assume that only babies need their full, undivided attention. But parents of older children must not underestimate the value of their presence. At every stage of development, parents have to find ways to connect to their children. Even teens, who often rebuff parental overtures, need more of a sense of connectedness with parents.

Children want their time with parents to be less rushed and stressed. They want more time doing simple things together. That means giving a child your undivided attention, accepting negative and positive feelings, being patient with emotional demands, and expressing affection.

Staying tuned in to children is a challenge. Attending to a child in a calm, caring way can have a powerful therapeutic impact. Those quiet moments together can benefit parents, too. Children can provide an alternative focus and a relief from the stresses of the world.

Action Plan

If you think your children don't realize it when you're stressed, you're wrong. Even small children intuitively know when Mom and Dad are not smiling as much or are less emotionally available to them. In my opinion, a parent's greatest priority is to be emotionally and physically available during a child's formative years. The time goes by in a flash, and there are no second chances. Also, children often learn more by example than by words. The old adage that "actions speak louder than words" holds true here. Most times, children are not fooled when what you say doesn't jibe with what you do. Some of the things that can get in the way of your being available include your overall stress level, work, leisure pursuits, and significant symptoms from medical or psychological conditions.

One of the first things taught in medical school is when you encounter a stressful situation, take your own pulse first. Overstressed doctors will not make the best decisions, and neither will parents. So you may need to do a stress self-exam. Look at your own moods. How available have you been to your family? How well are you sleeping and eating? How have you been feeling physically? Look for red flags before they turn into problems. Some of those red flags may be: you realize that you've dropped some weight; your kids say you're never home; or friends or coworkers say you look drawn and ask whether you're getting enough rest.

Part of the stress self-assessment should involve continuing medical care. Regular doctor visits are important, and are essential when parents get into their forties. Simple checkups and tests can find "red flags," signs of a brewing problem or indicate something that might go wrong in the future. So have your blood pressure and cholesterol levels checked; discuss your weight and diet with your doctor; have a stool test for hidden blood to detect colon cancer, and do a breast self-exam if you are a woman and have your prostate examined if you are a man to detect early signs of cancer. Colonoscopies are recommended for men over forty-five, and yearly mammograms for women over forty.

Another part of the stress self-exam should be a look at how well you are eating and sleeping, and whether you're getting enough exercise. People who eat regular meals and get regular amounts of sleep are, in general, less likely to succumb to the ravages of stress. Clearly, exercise helps you lose weight, sleep better, and reduce stress, possibly by raising levels of endorphins, the chemicals in the brain that lead to a natural high. Exercise also helps you feel calmer, stay younger, and sets a good example for your children. A sleepless, stressed-out existence not only is bad for your health but also sets a bad example for your children, since children tend to model their identities after their parents.

Take a moment to reflect on the amount of time you spend with your children. When was the last time you picked them up from school; went to one of their athletic events, recreational activities, or a school function; put them to bed; or sat down and had a meal with them? If may have been a while. Children are children only once. Your presence is important to their development. I believe that nothing at work matches the importance of being a presence in your child's life.

Making changes that will benefit your child is not as complicated as you would think. Try to get home a little earlier a few nights a week or make one practice session or a school function. Don't be afraid to tell colleagues that you need to get home on a particular day. Learn to say "no" to things that aren't absolutely essential to free some time for your children. While I was writing this book, another publisher asked me to write a chapter in a psychiatric book. It might have added another line to my resume, but when it came down to it, I decided that it would impose on my time with my children, so I declined the offer. We, as parents, have to make decisions like this all of the time. Such is life.

It's a delicate balance that leaves many parents feeling guilty about "not being there" for their children. Young children will always prefer your presence over someone else's. But you can't be there every second of every waking hour. All you can do is consistently monitor your involvement and occasionally stop and ask yourself, "How could I be with my children more?"

One way to answer that question is to schedule time to do things with your children. I take martial arts with my children several nights a week. Sports, yoga, and music are good outlets for spending time with your children. Or volunteer together. I have a friend who stays with her teenage son overnight at a soup kitchen once a month. Check with your church or synagogue for opportunities to volunteer as a family. Why wait until you're dissatisfied? Find time to do something that's helpful for others now.

If your life is stressful, then you need to address the stress. An important way to reduce stress is to set aside time for yourself, which may take some coordination with your spouse. My wife takes our children to piano lessons on Saturday morning, so that's when I go out for a long bike ride. Then I usually stay with them on Saturday afternoon, giving her some free time. I do most of my exercise either early in the morning or at night when my children are asleep. Some mornings, my wife goes to her spinning class before work and I get the children ready for school. Single parents have it tougher, and sometimes have to recruit friends and relatives to help out, or use babysitters. Everybody's got to have something that's relaxing, whether it's yoga, meditation, golf, a walk in the park, reading a good book, or watching an interesting movie. You can't ignore your need for time to relax and reflect. Again, you have to try to balance your personal needs and your children's needs.

I know one mother who, as a triathlete, trains up to six hours a day in addition to her full-time job, and rarely has any time for her child. Ask yourself, "Am I spending too much time by myself and not enough with my children?" Listen to what your children are saying to you about your leisure pursuits, and, if necessary, adjust accordingly. Your child's school play may take on more importance than taking a run that night.

Also, make more time for you and your spouse to be alone without any children. Hire a baby sitter to give you a child-free night, or send them to a friend's or family member's house for a few hours. Look at the stress of your marriage, which affects children on multiple levels. Ask yourself, "How much quality time do I have with my spouse?" "When was the last time we had dinner on our own?" "When was the last time we went away together on our own?" "How often have we been intimate?" "How well do we communicate, share household responsibilities in a mutually acceptable way, pinch-hit for one another, or give each other breaks?" The stresses of marriage, the stresses of each individual parent, and the stresses of the family all can affect how stressed your child is.

Parents need to work together to reduce their own stress. When our children were infants, I remember telling my wife, "You're exhausted. Time for you to take a nap. I'll take care of the babies." Parents of older children need to continue to nurture each other even when it's not so obvious that one or the other is physically or emotionally spent. Good parenting teammates let each other know when it's time for a break.

If you see stress in your spouse, you may need to help him or her first recognize and then deal with it. Deliver the message in a sensitive way by pointing to examples of why you believe your spouse is under stress. Provide objective observations without a critical edge and without blame, but with concern. If you deem the stress to be more dramatic, you may need to seek a psychological evaluation, particularly if you or your spouse has a family history of depression. Let's say your spouse's father got depressed in his forties. Now his son, your husband, is exhibiting signs of depression in his forties that affect his ability to interact with his children. He may need more than just a stress self-exam, perhaps a professional evaluation. You could discuss your concern with your doctor first. More tools are now available for primary care doctors to help them recognize stress and depression. With your doctor's help, you may be able to get a handle on the situation. If either you or your spouse is really anxious or depressed, then you may need a consultation with a mental health professional.

Action Points

1. Children know when you're stressed, even without them saying so.
2. Do a stress self-exam and notice any red flags that indicate you are stressed.
3. Maintain a healthy lifestyle to protect yourself from stress.
4. Make sure you spend time with your children.
5. Find time for yourself and for you and your spouse away from your children.
6. If you or your spouse is under stress, consider seeking help to get it under control.

CHAPTER 14

Recognizing Stress
in Children

$\int$ ome children handle stress better than others. Parents need to know their children's temperaments, which includes how resilient they are; the quality of their moods in general; how active they are physically; how they respond to new situations; and whether they need a lot—or very little—stimulation. Other things that affect how children respond to stress include illness, developmental level, conditioning, and getting enough rest.

This chapter shows parents how to find out their child's stress style using a stress analysis of the things that might be affecting their child. If there are numerous stressors in your child's life, he or she may be at risk for developing physical symptoms.

Common Behavioral Signals

While each child reacts differently to stress, some common behaviors, such as change in appetite, sleeplessness, headaches, or stomachaches my indicate moderate stress. Agitation, aggression, and withdrawal may signal more severe stress.

Reactions to stress may also manifest itself as a true psychiatric disorder. In general, anxiety is the most common response to extreme stress. Whether your child has a constellation of symptoms that fit a diagnostic category is a matter of degree. With enough distress and impairment, your child may quality for a diagnosis of a disorder. Some things to look for are how long the stress been going on and whether the stress significantly affects your child's ability to function. Stress for two weeks or longer or stress that affects two domains of a child's life—both at home and at school, for example—may signify significant stress. Also, you may recognize signs of significant stress that have led to bigger problems, such as anxiety or depression, in the past or in an older child or someone else in the family. Look for stress signs that fit a family pattern.

You needn't make your own diagnosis of a disorder before you get help. In fact, you may be misled by symptoms that look like something serious, but may not be. Your child may seem to be tired, have difficulty focusing attention, and be irritable, impulsive, and easily frustrated. These symptoms may resemble attention deficit hyperactivity disorder, but research shows that children who are sleep deprived may also have problems with attention and activity level. Your pediatrician is usually a good first choice to help evaluate your child's stress. Your doctor may have some suggestions for the family on how to deal with the stress before needing to refer you to a mental health professional.

Stress Makers

Parents can get a quick read on their child's stress level by looking at the potential sources of stress on the following Stress Makers Checklist. They can then look at the Stress Breakers Checklist (Chapter 15) to find ways to help neutralize stress.

The Stress Makers Checklist has some common sense items, but you may be surprised by some of the stressors listed. The checklist provides a global view of stress. You'll see that stress can be found in all of the domains—family, school, and home environment.

Stress Makers Checklist

❑ Changes in routine
❑ Overscheduling
❑ Too much emphasis on achievement
❑ Unreasonable expectations by parents
❑ Not playing enough with friends

- ☐ Illness in the child or a family member
- ☐ Divorce
- ☐ Moving
- ☐ Birth of a sibling
- ☐ Death of a family member or a pet
- ☐ Change of school
- ☐ Conflicts during meal times
- ☐ Not enough time spent with parents
- ☐ Poor parent-child communication
- ☐ Inconsistent discipline by parents
- ☐ Sleep problems
- ☐ Remarriage of a parent
- ☐ Learning disabilities or academic problems
- ☐ Social problems
- ☐ Problems with a teacher
- ☐ Conflict with family members
- ☐ Separation from a parent
- ☐ Going on an overnight trip away from parents
- ☐ Physically developing relatively early or late
- ☐ Not being good at sports (especially for boys)
- ☐ Being overweight

Stress and the Body

Your mental state can affect your physical health. As mentioned earlier, stress causes changes in the immune system and can affect health negatively. Stress triggers a number of biochemical changes in the body, and can affect heart function, hormone levels, the nervous system, and metabolic rates. Psychoneuroimmunologists have concluded that stress appears to be the common denominator of many illnesses ranging from the common cold to heart disease and cancer.

Stress can help children sculpt their strengths and abilities, just as a weightlifters use weights to sculpt their muscles. Adding on more weight, little by little, allows weightlifters to increase strength because they learn how to handle the added load. Too much weight on one side of the barbell and they topple over, and may even injure themselves. The same goes for stress—when children learn how to handle it a little at a time their ability to master new, challenging situations grows. Parents who can recognize the stresses their children are exposed to and determine whether they will be overwhelmed can help promote healthy coping strategies by teaching and modeling.

Action Plan

You can estimate the level of your child's stress by looking at his or her reactions to stress. Stress itself is not bad. It's all a matter of degree. The type and degree of stress will affect whether it has a negative impact on your child or makes your child stronger. Just as children can build up immunities by being exposed to infections, they can learn to develop the ability to deal with stress. In other words, if your child was never exposed to any bacteria or viruses, then the child's immune system would never develop, and exposure to an infection might result in a severe illness. Similarly, shielding your child from all stress will not prepare the child to get through the inevitable stresses of life. Some stresses, however, are off the chart, such as child abuse, and a child should, of course, be protected from them.

Listen to your child, watch, and then try to figure out at what point he or she seems to be overwhelmed. For example, when teaching your child to swim, you must let go gradually. A child needs to slowly build up the skill and swimming muscles to be able to swim unsupported. You watch and see when you may need to grab your child because it looks like he or she is starting to sink. Then, at some point, he or she is working hard but will make it to the other side of the pool. It's a judgment call. Children need the freedom to do as much as they can on their own in a gradual way as they grow up, even if it's stressful. So don't be too quick to jump in to protect your child from stress. It's not realistic or practical, and not good for your child. Also, as children get older and acquire more life experience, they tend to manage stressful situations more easily. Watch them, guide them, and protect them, but try to help them fight their own battles.

Sometimes, something that had not been stressful at one point in a child's life may become stressful later, or during a specific situation. For example, if your child has a cold, a physically stressful situation, such as a sports tryout in the middle of exam week, may be too much to bear. Susceptibility to stress is somewhat like susceptibility to infection. If your children get run down, they may become more susceptible to the effects of stress. One child who deals well with change might not be fazed by going to a new summer camp, while another who abides by a set routine may become stressed at going to camp. As parents, you need to ask: What kind of a child do I have? Stress is not necessarily an either-or issue, but ebbs and flows, depending on the situation.

Another question you may ask to find out the dynamic effects of stress on your child is whether significant stresses are coming from a variety of sources at once. For example, a parent may be ill at the same time as your child is having problems with a teacher and also squabbling with a best friend. A combination of stresses all at once, like having more than one infection at the same time, can overload a child.

You can also point out examples of stress to your child when you see it. Look at how New York Yankees' pitcher Roger Clemens dealt with the stress of pitching in a World Series game—by throwing a broken bat at the New York Mets's Mike Piazza. I made sure to tell my son that that was not a good way to deal with stress.

Be sure to compliment your children when they do something well, such as, "I like the way you did your homework assignment two days in advance. Now you have the whole weekend free." "I saw you practicing for your recital. Now you'll really be prepared for it." Without even knowing it, you model how to handle stress all of the time. When you drop something on the floor, do you curse under your breath, or do you say, "That's not a good move," and calmly clean it up. Practice good stress hygiene yourself and compliment your children when they do, too, and everyone will be less stressful.

Action Points

1. Look at your child's reactions to stress carefully.
2. Try to get a feel for when your child is overwhelmed by stress.
3. Don't be too protective of stress. Let your child slowly develop an ability and personal style for dealing with his or her own stress.
4. Be aware that stress ebbs and flows, depending on the situation.
5. Look for a combination of stresses from different sources.
6. Be a model for good stress behavior, and compliment your children when they handle stress well.

PART III

Helping

Your Child

Feel Better

CHAPTER 15

Calming Your Child—
Stress Antidotes

*M*y oldest girl, Carly, age ten, was nervous and not sleeping well the week before she was to go to overnight camp for the first time. When I brought up camp in conversation, she became upset. So I asked her what she was feeling about camp, and she said, "I'm afraid I'll miss you and Mommy."

I told her honestly, "You will miss us a lot the first few days." So we talked about what she could do to lessen the stress of being away from home. She decided to take along a picture of our family, to write us post-cards, and to distract herself with camp activities. Though I generally dislike hand-held computer games, I got her one to pass the time and help distract her when she was homesick.

Translation: "I'm scared about being away from home, and I don't know how to handle it."

Children lean on their parents, siblings, and friends to learn how to handle stress. Parents can help their children cope when they recognize the first signs that the stress balance is beginning to tip, and then know what to do. Children's natural reaction to overly stressful situations is to avoid them or deny them. Through rehearsal and coaching from parents, children can learn more active ways to manage stress. Children also learn by watching role models, specifically their parent's example. Parents should remember that children listen to what they say, and, maybe more importantly, watch what they do. This chapter shares what I have learned in years of parenting and working with children to reduce the stresses of childhood.

Parents Can Make a Difference

Parents are in the best position to provide a supportive environment, help set priorities, and encourage the development of healthy stress-relieving habits in their children. Athletes take a break when they alternate a hard training day with an easy one. Recovery from stress, which includes rest and good nutrition, is essential for children as well.

Children often make comments about how they feel at the moment, but make it sound as if they always feel that way. Just listen, and maybe point out to the child that she didn't feel that "life sucks" last week. Try to find out what's on the child's mind at that moment. Then work together to come up with a strategy to deal with it.

I disagree with the popular psychology that says it doesn't matter what parents do because everything is based on genetics. Genes are important, but they are not everything. What's generally inherited is a predisposition toward a problem. The actual expression of the genes involved is a combination of nature and nurture. Even identical twins have different types of illnesses and different personalities.

So don't abdicate the parental throne or go on parental autopilot. You have important work to do. You can't just assume that everything is predetermined if you don't get immediate results in helping to defuse stress. A parent who thinks a child is difficult and doesn't listen may try everything and just give up because that's the way the child is. In most cases, children don't change their behavior based on being told something once or twice. They change as they grow. Just as a flower turns toward the sun as it grows, dealing with the stresses of growing up is a gradual process. You have to shape behavior over time.

Stress Breakers

Parents may use the following Stress Breakers Checklist to help their children build a tool kit for combating stress. The idea behind stress breaking is to hit stress from a lot of directions. It's also important to allow children plenty of unstructured time just to goof off and relax. Simple relaxation techniques and biofeedback can also help children learn to cope with stress. Karen Olness's studies show that children can be hypnotized into boosting their immune systems and can actually decrease the incidence of upper respiratory infections; in her study, the children actually were hypnotized to increase the amount of immunoglobulins in their saliva!

Stress Breakers Checklist

- ☐ Acceptance and understanding by parents
- ☐ Friendships
- ☐ Quality time with parents
- ☐ Sports
- ☐ Listening to music
- ☐ Movies
- ☐ Being read to by a parent
- ☐ Reading to a parent
- ☐ Adequate sleep and nutrition
- ☐ Creative play
- ☐ Writing, drawing, or other relaxing projects
- ☐ Being outside
- ☐ Telling jokes
- ☐ Laughing
- ☐ Taking care of pets

Family fun-time activities can be great stress breakers. A family can read a favorite story together, look at family pictures, make popcorn, or go to the zoo, a museum, or a sporting event. Walking regularly, like most physical exercise, not only helps relieve pent-up tension but also prevents stress buildup, both for parents and children.

When you think about specific stress-breaking techniques, think broadly. Some children don't go for formalized treatment, such as biofeedback. Others really enjoy that. Tailor what you do to your own child's preferences.

I often liken a child's overall stress level to the tide. When it's high, a small storm may cause flooding. If it's low, then even a good-sized storm may be easily absorbed by the land. General diversions that keep kids relaxed—being read to, reading to a parent, creative play—help to keep the stress tide way out to sea.

Play is an important way that children work out their conflicts and what's on their minds. It helps to both diffuse stress and act as a diversion. When my young patients are about to have an operation, I routinely give them a dollhouse and toys, often with some medical props, and give them a chance to play out some of their fears in the more controlled setting of play.

Writing, drawing, and other more organized projects diffuse stress by distraction. They also help the child relate to what's going on in a more free-form way.

Exercise is a great stress reducer, even for children. Play an active game of catch, shoot baskets, or go bike riding. Do whatever your child likes to do, but do it together.

One of my favorite ways to diffuse stress is through humor. Telling jokes and laughing can change a child's mood and dissolve stress almost immediately. Making light of a situation helps point out when a child may be overreacting. My six-year-old son Zach said he was afraid of getting hit in the head by the ball when he was up at bat. So I told him, "The pitcher isn't throwing hard enough to hurt you, especially since you're wearing a helmet. And even if you did get hit, it wouldn't be so bad— you'd get to go to first base!"

Try to stay lighthearted when stressful situations come up. And don't let your own stress get in the way. When my daughter Carly said she was nervous about going to overnight camp for the first time, I didn't tell her that my wife and I were even more nervous about having our first-born being away for the whole summer. I tried hard not to let her know that, and put on a happy face whenever we talked about camp. I emphasized how much fun she was going to have and all of the neat things she could take with her. And we all made it through the summer without incident.

Internal and External Stress

As we discussed in the previous chapter, stress may come from many sources either internal—from within the child—or external—from the outside world. Internal stresses often become manifested by changes in sleep, mood, and eating habits, or destructive behaviors such as alcohol or drug use in adolescents. External stresses may come from what's going on in school, or bullies, teachers, or whatever you believe may be influencing your child, and may lead to anxiety or depressed mood.

For internal stress, techniques such as distraction, listening to music, reading, or playing computer games often help. Watch Olympic athletes as they prepare to compete and you'll notice that many of them wear headphones. Listening to music helps distract them as they psych themselves up for a very stressful event. They also make sure to get adequate amounts of sleep and to eat right to help shore up their bodies. Your child may not face Olympic-sized stress, but you can have stress-reduction tools at your disposable and make sure that your child is in good physical shape to face the stresses of life.

For your child's external stress, you may need to intervene to help relieve the stress. If your child is being bullied, call the bully's parent and teacher to discuss the situation. (For more on how to handle bullies, see Chapter 9.) Similarly, if your child is having difficulty with a specific subject, call the teacher and ask for specific help. If a child can't finish a school assignment, and needs an extension, talk to the teacher, or have the child approach the teacher. Children tend to think in extremes. They also often misinterpret situations and don't know how to read adults. You can help cut through a child's misinterpretation that the teacher "hates" the child, or won't be receptive to talking to him or her. Part of your job as a parent is to help your child better understand adults and to clarify when an adult is truly unhappy.

Most parents know just by looking at a child's reaction that the child is upset. Sometimes a little emotional stroking can diffuse stress. A carefully placed pat on the back, either physically or verbally, can go a long way to relieving stress.

Empower Children

Children need to be able to do something to handle their stress and to feel more in control of a world, which they may find frightening. Such actions may be giving a young child a misting bottle filled with water as a "monster repellent" to be sprayed under the bed or helping an older child through a self-hypnosis exercise when that uh-oh feeling in the stomach comes on.

A neat way to introduce children to stress reduction is through audiotapes. These tapes typically tell an enchanting tale for children of all ages and go through a guided imagery relaxation journey, inviting children to use their imaginations to create a beautiful resting place of their own.

You can help your kids succeed by loading the stress seesaw so it's always tipping in their favor. Success breeds success, and that carries over to other situations. When you empower your children, and they do well, they are more confident and more likely to succeed later on in other endeavors.

Self-Hypnosis

Hypnosis in children is somewhat different from hypnosis in adults. Many children can shift easily from one cognitive state to another and can rapidly enter into a "hypnotic" state, which is similar to the mesmerizing feeling you get sometimes while driving a long distance on a highway, when you may lose track of time, which is a state of relaxed distraction.

The hypnotic state is analogous to pretending, daydreaming, imagining, or being fully absorbed in an activity, such as reading a good book, watching a television show, or attending a concert. When you help a tired infant fall asleep, you're using your natural ability to induce hypnosis. Some successful teachers and coaches develop this ability as they fine-tune their communication skills with children.

You can help a child use imagery or distraction as a hypnotic technique or remind an older child to use self-hypnosis to deal with stress or prevent it. One of the misconceptions about hypnosis is that the person performing hypnosis, called a hypnotherapist, possesses some magical powers. Actually, the patient is the hypnotherapist, and the therapist's or parent's role is that of coach or guide.

Hypnotherapy—the use of hypnosis as a therapeutic adjunct—has been shown to be useful in a wide variety of childhood problems, including bed wetting, insomnia, migraine headaches, nail biting, sleepwalking, tics, hair pulling, as well as in drug abuse, obesity, and phobias.

The techniques used for children vary according to their developmental stage and age. Children of all ages have demonstrated the ability to alter sensation, perceptions, and experience. Young children under age six who at times have blurred boundaries between reality and fantasy may enter hypnosis easily, but may move in and out and back into the hypnotic state rapidly and repeatedly. They may not show the typical behaviors of adults—relaxed muscles and closed eyes. Instead, a young, hypnotized child may have wide open eyes and move around a bit.

While younger children have little difficulty using their imaginations during hypnosis, teens tend to have fewer spontaneous images, learn relaxation somewhat more slowly, and are less adept at controlling their mind/body state. Even so, teens, like adults, can learn and master self-hypnosis techniques when they are motivated to change. They must learn to trust the person, be it a therapist or parent, who can teach and guide them in the proper technique.

Relaxation in School

School programs across the country now use relaxation techniques such as deep breathing, guided imagery, yoga, and acupressure. In Michigan, a health education plan has taught students to breathe deeply to help them relax and think clearly. In Minnesota, teachers lead students on "imagery trips" to reduce stress. In California, stress-reduction programs including yoga and acupressure have received widespread support from parents and school administrators.

Relaxation programs in school are important because students are under far more stress today. When teachers in the 1940s talked about students' problems, they meant running in the hallways and chewing gum. Now, teachers worry about students taking drugs, not being supervised by parents, and causing or becoming victims of violence.

Schools in general are paying more attention to emotional health than they used to. Teachers attend workshops on social and emotional learning and receive orientation to address their students' emotional needs, which will help them reduce students' stress.

Taming Test Anxiety

Parents can help tame test anxiety in their school-aged children by recognizing the problem and reinforcing realistic expectations. For example, it's good to note that one test usually doesn't count for an entire grade.

I can't emphasize enough the importance of preparation. Being pre-pared is the biggest issue surrounding test anxiety. A baseball player puts his best swing into unconscious memory by taking batting practice for hours at a time so he can handle wicked curve balls. Test anxiety is like stepping up to the plate. Students want to prepare and rehearse as much as possible so that their instincts take over. Then when they finally sit down to take the tests, they'll be much less susceptible to anxiety.

The more closely you can help your child replicate the testing situa-tion, the better the chances of heading off test anxiety. Scholastic Aptitude Test (SAT) preparation courses are so popular, and so successful, because they have students take sample tests over and over again. Not only do the students learn how to take the SAT, they practice taking the test under realistic conditions, in a quiet room with a timed deadline. Again, prepa-ration is the key.

When the teacher says, "Now, begin," the best anxiety reliever is deep breathing. I teach children to take deep, rhythmic breaths through the nose and imagine they are blowing up a balloon in the belly. Once the balloon is fully inflated, they hold their breathe for a second or two, then release. As they exhale, I suggest they try to relax all of their mus-cles. I say, "Breathe in slowly to a count of three, and exhale to a count of six." For younger children, I use a different visual image, suggesting they make their bodies like Raggedy Anne, limp spaghetti, or a bowl of Jell-O. The goal is simply to be loose.

A tip for students to avoid freezing up during an exam is: skip over difficult sections and answer the questions you know to get your confi-dence level up, then go back to the difficult sections. To go back to the Olympic athletes for a moment, if they make a mistake during an event, say in ice skating, they push on and finish the rest of the program. The same holds true for test taking. Don't let a mistake in one part affect the rest of the test. I tell my patients, "If you have difficulty in one section, you may still salvage a good grade if you ace the rest of it. So if you're having difficulty, go on to something else and don't dwell on it."

Another testing-taking tip is: take a break—get a glass of water or wash your face. Sometimes students can't remember details because they're thinking too hard. In most real-life situations, you can take a moment to collect yourself. If necessary, be like a baseball player and step out of the batter's box for a moment. A minibreak may be just what's needed for the answers to come to mind.

If students don't understand a question, they shouldn't be afraid to ask for help. The worst thing that can happen is the teacher will say, "I can't help you."

One final tip: have your child draw on experiences where he or she was called upon to produce on the spot. I think it's great for children to perform in plays, recitals, and organized sports in front of people at any early age. This experience helps them get used to the pressure of performing in front on an audience. This boost in confidence they get from performing well carries over into similar pressure-packed situations, including test taking. You might say to a nervous child the night before a test, "Remember how nervous you were about your dance recital last year. But you practiced a lot, and when the music started, you took a few deep breaths, and you were great." Similarly, you might say, "Remember your dance recital when you made a small mistake at the beginning of the program, which no one in the audience even noticed, and after that, it went fine."

Ringing in the Holidays

Holidays are a wonderful time of year. As they grow nearer, though, the events of the season often change from cheerful to stressful ones for families, especially children. Parents need to take a close look at how the family manages holidays. If parents are aware of their child's stress indicators, it may be possible to avoid many of them and experience a happy holiday season.

Parents may feel more stress than their children during the holidays. As I've mentioned, if you're stressed-out, then your children will likely pick up on it and may become stressed as well. Also, having more family and friends around is not necessarily what makes children happy. For children, that means sharing their parents, and they often lose out if their parents are wrapped up in spending time with relatives and friends. Try to make sure to set aside time for yourself to catch up with friends and relatives, but also leave some quality time for your children. Holidays should be a time to reconnect with everyone in the family. Don't let your children get lost in the hustle and bustle of holidays.

Action Plan

Once you've recognized your child is under stress, you can learn to divert, diffuse, or delay the stress. Divert means to redirect the stress to help your child get out of its way. See whether you can change the situation slightly so that stress doesn't hit as hard. If the stress is unavoidable, try to expose your child to it in a less vulnerable way. Diffuse means to advise your child on how to best deal with the situation. If your child is involved in a stressful conflict, talk it out with your child. Delay means to postpone the stress, if possible, so that your child has more time to deal with it, such as getting an extension on a term paper.

You may have to simply avoid the stress. Maybe a young child shouldn't go to a relative's funeral. For a sick child, a parent should stay overnight in the hospital with him or her.

You can help your child prepare for stressful situations. Preparation is like training, and strengthens your child to meet the challenge. For a young child, talk about visiting a place before you go there. Take your budding Little Leaguer to a batting cage before his baseball tryout. Help your teenager study the night before a big test. Perform the preparation as close to the real event as you can. For example, take your child to visit a new school or look at a camp video together just before starting school or camp.

Anytime you can, have your child use his or her imagination to rehearse a stressful situation. Rehearsing almost exactly the way it will happen can help reduce stress by preparing your child for the actual situation. You can even role-play with your child. If a friend hurt your child's feelings, tell her, "Okay, I'll be your friend. Tell me what you'd like to say to me." If your child is nervous about reading a poem in front of the class, have him make believe he's in the classroom, and have him read the poem to you.

Talk about what will probably happen, what's the worst that could happen, and let the stress come out. Then let your child come up with ways to lessen the stress, or make some general suggestions that lead your child to developing his or her own personal stress breakers. You might also talk about how you got through a stressful situation to help break the ice.

You don't necessarily have to talk about a stressful situation. More often than not, children choose not to acknowledge what's bothering them. When my wife took Carly to camp, instead of saying, "You'll probably be nervous during the car ride," I suggested that she take along her hand-held video game to play in the car. Parents may not need to bring the stress to a conscious level. If you know your child is under stress, and the child denies it, don't just give up because your child won't talk about it, or ignore it, thinking that your child must not be stressed-out. You can make a difference, without throwing the stress in your child's face. Address the underlying issue using stress breakers.

The good news is that it's unlikely that one mistake will destroy your child, so you can take chances. Even if you get things only partly right, and diffuse a little stress, that's okay. Twelve-year-old Josh was being sent to a residential school, but didn't want to talk to me about going away. I saw him for a good-bye visit the week he was to leave. A few days later, his mother called to say that Josh wanted to see me again. When he came in, I asked, "What's on your mind?"

He said, "Nothing."

I said he looked a little teary-eyed, and he said: "Allergies."

Then I asked him, "What's the longest time you've been away from home?" He told me, one week. Not knowing exactly where I was going, I thought maybe he wanted me to wish him good luck, to feel somehow connected with me. So we talked about how he'd probably miss his parents because he wouldn't see them for a few weeks and what he could do to feel less lonely, and we worked out contingency plans when that happened. I told him he could contact me, that I would always be his doctor, and that I would be in touch with the doctors at his new school. I probably got to the core issue, but even if I got to only half of what was on his mind, that was okay because Josh said he felt better after talking to me.

Another way to break a child's stress cycle is to get away from the family, even for a short time. Just as parents need a break from their children, children need a break from their parents. Have your child spend a day at a friend's house, go away for the weekend on a school trip, or spend quiet time in his or her room without any siblings or parents. This need applies to young children as well as teens.

Reading a book, doing a puzzle, or listening to music is important. Children need to be able to divert themselves without their parent's guidance, and to learn that it's okay to be alone. As children get older, they have to deal with being alone more and more. They need to know what they can do to pass the time while they wait for a parent to pick them up or during that first night of overnight camp. Parents can help children cultivate activities that divert, relax, and act as stress breakers.

Action Points

1. Divert, delay, or diffuse stress.
2. Help prepare your child for stressful situations.
3. Rehearse a stressful situation with your child, but don't throw the stress in the child's face.
4. Use Stress Breakers to address the underlying stress.
5. Allow your child to take a break, alone.
6. Help your child cultivate activities that divert and relieve stress.

CHAPTER 16

Mixing in Medications

The news media pegged it a sharp rise in psychiatric drugs for the young, citing troubling reports that school-age—and younger—children were taking more stimulants, antidepressants, and other psychiatric drugs. But in fact this study of data on attention deficit hyperactivity disorder (ADHD) released in February 2000 was based on drugs prescribed for preschoolers in two specific populations. The study did not include information about the children's diagnoses or about whether primary care physicians or specialists prescribed the drugs. And the authors, led by University of Maryland's Julie Zito, Ph.D., could not determine whether the children received comprehensive therapy, including behavioral interventions, or just a drug.

Politicians have seized the opportunity to condemn "overmedicating" youngsters. Diagnoses such as ADHD and depression have become increasingly popular, which puts pressure on parents to do something for their children. In many cases, drugs are given as a last resort, prescribed in the hope of protecting the child's safety, ensuring the safety of others, or offering relief to a child whose life is being swallowed up by symptoms.

This chapter lays out the various types of drugs prescribed by physicians, including a table listing medications, conditions treated, proper dosing, and side effects. It also delves into the issues of which drugs are appropriate, and when. Some family doctors are making diagnoses based on symptom checklists rather than on a thorough evaluation of a child's life, both in and out of the home. This diagnostic style may lead to quick, inexpensive pharmacological fixes instead of a therapy specifically designed for the child's condition. The American Academy of Pediatrics just released its first-ever hyperactivity guidelines to help doctors better identify youngsters with the problem while preventing children who are just rambunctious from being medicated. Timely evaluation and proper treatment can reduce the risks for school failure and dropout, as well as drug abuse and stunted physical, emotional, social, and intellectual development.

Using Medications

Medication can be an effective part of a child's treatment plan. A doctor's recommendation to use medication often brings up questions and concerns, by you and your child. Any doctor who recommends medication should have experience in treating childhood or adolescent psychiatric illnesses. You should receive a full explanation about the reasons for using medication, the medication's benefits as well as unwanted side effects or dangers, and other treatment alternatives.

Before taking a psychiatric drug, a child should have an evaluation by a pediatrician and have appropriate consultations. As I've pointed out, many medical conditions can present as psychiatric conditions. Psychiatric medication should be used as part of a comprehensive treatment plan, which usually includes individual or family psychotherapy and a parent's guidance. You may need to adjust the medication doses or use additional medications to best meet your child's needs. Since side effects may range from the simply annoying to the very serious, and each child reacts differently to medications, you also need to stay in close contact with your doctor. Don't stop or change any medication without first consulting with the doctor.

Before recommending any medication, a child psychiatrist will usually interview the child and do a thorough diagnostic evaluation, according to the American Academy of Child and Adolescent Psychiatry. This may include a physical exam, psychological testing, laboratory tests, other medical tests such as an electrocardiogram (EKG) or electroencephalogram (EEG), and consultation with other medical specialists, such as neurologists.

When appropriately prescribed and taken as directed, medication may reduce or eliminate troubling symptoms and improve your child's daily functioning. Your child should be included in discussions about medications, discussions that are conducted in child-friendly language.

If you still have serious questions or doubts about medication, ask for a second opinion by a child and adolescent psychiatrist. Parents seeking a referral to a local child and adolescent psychiatrist may contact the AACAP, 3615 Wisconsin Avenue, NW, Washington, D.C. 20016, (202) 966-7300, or visit the Web site at *www.aacap.org.*

Medication Plus Behavioral Therapy for ADHD

As an example of how medication can, and should, be combined with other therapies, let's look at ADHD. Current ADHD treatment includes a mix of approaches, such as drug therapy, counseling, and supportive services in schools and communities. The medical literature offers many studies carried out over brief treatment periods (three months or less). To get an idea of the best ADHD treatment in the long run, the National Institute of Mental Health (NIMH) sponsored an ongoing, multisite, treatment study of children with ADHD, entitled "The Multimodal Treatment Study of Children with Attention Deficit Hyperactivity Disorder (MTA)."

MTA brought together eighteen nationally recognized authorities in ADHD at six different university medical centers and hospitals to evaluate the leading treatments for ADHD, including various forms of behavior therapy and medications. The study included nearly 600 elementary school children, ages seven to nine, randomly assigned to one of four treatment groups: medication alone, psychosocial/behavioral treatment alone, a combination of the two, or routine community care.

The first MTA results by lead author Peter Jensen, M.D., a Columbia University psychiatrist, indicate that long-term combination treatments and medication management alone are both significantly superior to intensive behavioral treatments and routine community treatments in reducing ADHD symptoms for up to fourteen months. The combined treatment approach was consistently superior to routine community care, specifically in anxiety symptoms, academic performance, oppositional behavior, parent-child relations, and social skills. On the other hand, the single medication-only or behavioral-only treatments were not superior. In addition, the combined treatment allowed children to take somewhat lower doses of medication, compared to the medication-only group.

The MTA study demonstrates that, on average, carefully monitored medication management with monthly follow-up is more effective than intensive behavioral treatment for ADHD symptoms for as long as fourteen months. All of the children tended to improve, but those on careful medication management generally showed the greatest improvement. For important daily functioning, including academic performance and family relationships, the combination of medication and behavioral therapy produced improvements better than community care.

It's important to note that the children's families and teachers reported somewhat higher levels of satisfaction when behavioral therapy was included in treatment. So medication alone is not necessarily the best treatment for every child with ADHD, and families should pursue treatment that includes other therapies along with medication. In fact, the findings show that children with other accompanying problems, such as anxiety or high levels of family stress, seem to do best with approaches that combine medication and intensive behavioral therapy.

One of the surprise findings of the study was that children treated with effective medication management, either alone or in combination with behavioral therapy, showed substantially greater improvements in social skills and peer relationships than those in the community treatment group. This important finding indicates that ADHD symptoms may interfere with learning specific social skills. Effective medication management may help relieve symptoms that had interfered with the child's social development.

The study's overall results appear to apply to a wide range of children and families who must deal with ADHD. However, the quality and intensity of the medication treatments in the study were substantially better than what you could expect to receive in the real world. During the first month of treatment, the researchers took special care to find an optimal medication dose for each child receiving medication. Then the children were seen for a thirty-minute, monthly visit. During these visits, the doctor spoke with the parent, met with the child, and discussed any concerns they might have regarding the medication or the child's ADHD-related symptoms. If the child was experiencing any difficulties, the doctor would consider adjusting the child's medication rather than taking a "wait and see" approach. The goal was to obtain substantial benefit that left "no room for improvement" compared with the functioning of children who did not have ADHD. This close supervision also fostered early detection and treatment for any medication side effects, which may have helped the children remain on effective treatment. In addition, the study doctors sought input from the children's teachers each month, and factored this information into decisions on adjusting treatments.

While the study doctors in the medication-only group did not provide behavioral therapy, they did advise parents about any concerns parents brought up, and provided reading materials and additional information upon request. They generally prescribed three drug doses per day and somewhat higher doses of stimulant medications. In comparison, the community-treatment doctors generally saw the children face to face only once or twice a year for shorter in-office visits, did not have any interaction with teachers, and prescribed lower doses and twice-daily stimulant medication.

Landmark Studies

Several landmark studies have been published that show the safety and effectiveness of certain medications for children with mental disorders.

Up-to-date information on the safety and efficacy of medications for children and adolescents with mental disorders was presented in a comprehensive series of articles in the May 1999 issue of the *Journal of the American Academy of Child and Adolescent Psychiatry*. The articles indicated that the most widely prescribed psychotropic medications for children, stimulants and selective serotonin reuptake inhibitors (SSRIs), are safe and effective in the short term for specific conditions, such as OCD.

There have been few systematic studies on the extent of use of all of the major classes of psychoactive medications for children and adolescents. Previous studies had been conducted by a single institution, or had focused on a single medication, such as methylphenidate (Ritalin) for ADHD. To address this gap, a team from the NIMH analyzed prescribing patterns and drug safety for children younger than eighteen by examining data from the National Ambulatory Medical Care Survey. This is an annual survey conducted by the federal government's National Center for Health Statistics, and the National Disease and Therapeutic Index, a pharmaceutical marketing database.

For the first time ever, the researchers assembled the latest information on the actual level of all psychoactive medication prescriptions for children, combined these data with current evidence of safety and efficacy, and identified mismatches between clinical practices and scientific evidence. Expert investigators across the United States compiled evidence on the safety and efficacy of the entire range of psychoactive medications prescribed for American children and adolescents and made recommendations for future studies.

The data focused on children's visits to physicians for psychiatric reasons involving a prescription for a psychotropic medication. The results from the consensus review show good support for the safety and short-term efficacy of stimulants, which were prescribed most to treat ADHD, and for SSRIs, the second most prescribed group of agents, to treat major depression and OCD. Tricyclic antidepressants (TCAs) were the third most frequently mentioned, and central adrenergic agonists, such as clonidine, used to treat sleep disturbances in ADHD, ranked fourth.

The team suggested that the federal researchers in this area should target the development of short-term safety and efficacy studies of medications where knowledge is limited, levels of prescribing are highest, and potential for toxicities with long-term exposure are most prominent.

Another important NIMH-funded study found that the SSRI fluvoxamine is, indeed, an effective treatment for anxiety disorders. The multisite study, involving 128 children and adolescents, ages six to seventeen, found that the medication was more than twice as effective as the placebo over an eight-week period. Symptoms improved in 76 percent of the sixty-three children randomly assigned to the antidepressant drug compared to only 29 percent of the sixty-five children assigned to the placebo group, according to the study, which was published in the *New England Journal of Medicine* in April 2001.

There were no severe side effects from the medication. The children on fluvoxamine and those on the placebo had some side effects, which were usually mild. Only stomachache was more frequent among the children on fluvoxamine (49 percent) than those on the placebo (28 percent). Those taking the medication also showed greater increases in activity levels than those in the placebo group. Only five of the sixty-three children in the medication group discontinued treatment as a result of side effects, compared with one of the sixty-five children in the placebo group.

Why is the study important? It is the first placebo-controlled, multisite study of an SSRI in children and adolescents with anxiety disorders. Anxiety disorders often go unrecognized, and untreated, and can cause significant suffering and functional impairment if left untreated. While not all children will continue to suffer anxiety disorders as adults, some will, and early treatment may help prevent future problems such as depression and suicide. Knowing that there is an effective medical treatment will, I hope, get more anxious children the treatment they need.

The children in this study needed to have at least one of these anxiety disorders in order to participate: generalized anxiety disorder, separation anxiety disorder, or social phobia. These disorders are generally recognized through a careful evaluation, usually by a child psychiatrist, that includes examining the child, taking a medical history, and interviewing the child's parents. For this study, the children and adolescents had to go through an additional extended evaluation that lasted three weeks and included psychotherapy. Only those children who did not improve with psychotherapy alone were entered into the medication study. That avoided exposing children to medications when simple support and encouragement might have been enough to ease their anxiety.

The results do not imply that anxious children should be treated with medications alone. In fact, one specific form of psychotherapy, cognitive behavioral therapy (CBT), is the recommended treatment for children with anxiety disorders, according to the Child Academy. The success of CBT has been documented in research. Temple University researchers led by P. Kendall have found that CBT was an effective treatment for 173 children, ages eight to thirteen, with a variety of anxiety disorders. Others have found CBT may be a useful treatment for social phobia and OCD.

Two other landmark studies involving SSRIs also deserve notice. The first is a fluoxetine study led by Dallas psychiatrist Graham Emslie, M.D., which was the first to show any antidepressant was effective for pediatric depression. The second is a more recent study led by Brown University psychiatrist M. Keller that shows the effectiveness of paroxetine in the treatment of teens with major depression.

A Treatment Plan

Once parents have recognized symptoms and sought medical help, they should discuss a treatment plan with the child's physician, which may include medications. Medications may enhance psychotherapy, family therapy, and school consultation as part of a child's comprehensive treatment. Medications should: not automatically be considered the first treatment choice; not be used alone; and be used only when their benefits outweigh the risks. I suggest a trial period of three to four weeks of other interventions without medications before you consider starting medications.

Parents must also monitor medications closely. Careful observation helps ensure that your child is getting the appropriate dosage. Talk to your psychiatrist about all medications your child is taking, including nonprescription medicines, to learn of possible complications or interactions.

Other treatment plan suggestions include:

- Talk regularly with your child's teachers, caregivers, and physicians about how your child is doing, especially when medication is first started, restarted, or when the dose is changed.
- Applaud your child for improvements in behavior (getting better grades, developing social skills, having more friends). The therapy and medications are not responsible for these improvements—they simply make it possible for your child's assets and natural skills to shine through.
- Find a school or classroom setting that can provide structure and organization beneficial to your child. Your child does not need unnecessary pressure and inappropriate expectations.
- Help children feel comfortable with their therapy and medication and understand that treatment is usually a temporary situation. They need to know the value of their treatment program and that being a part of it does not make them different from the rest of their peers.

Medication Review

The next section reviews treatment with medications, providing extensive information regarding the complete range of treatment options. The following table tells you about each of these drugs, how they are used, and potential side effects.

Stimulants

Stimulants are by far the most widely researched and commonly prescribed treatments for children with ADHD. They diminish overactivity and impulsive behaviors seen in ADHD and allow the child to sustain attention and improve physical coordination (used in such activities as handwriting and sports). Use of stimulants can result in an immediate and often dramatic improvement in behavior both at school and at home. The benefits and the risks associated with stimulants must be weighed carefully, and evaluated and monitored continually. In general, stimulants are regarded as an effective, safe ADHD therapy with relatively few side effects.

More than 200 controlled studies of more than 6,000 children, most of them Caucasian boys, show that stimulants are effective for ADHD, including significant benefits for cognition and social function. Studies of stimulants show robust short-term results and a good safety profile. While there are few long-term studies in existence, there is no evidence that careful use of these drugs is harmful. The current evidence indicates that stimulants are safe and effective in studies lasting as long as two years.

A recent look at more than 1,000 young children with ADHD by Harvard psychiatrist Timothy Wilens, M.D., shows that they may be less likely to develop a substance-abuse disorder if they receive treatment with a stimulant such as methylphenidate. This finding is the opposite of some of the concerns about children being more at risk of substance abuse if they get stimulant treatment for ADHD. More research is needed to confirm the finding.

Examples include: methylphenidate (Ritalin), dextroamphetamine (Dexedrine), mixtures of dextroamphetamine salts (Adderall), and pemoline (Cylert). Please be aware that there have been warnings about liver failure associated with the use of Cylert, and, in my opinion, it should not be used for children.

Several once-daily methylphenate preparations have now been approved, including Concerta, Metadate CD, and Adderall XR, and others, including Ritalin LA (for long-acting), may soon be available. The trend is toward extended-release formulations because they have certain advantages. An ADHD child doesn't have to go to the school nurse at lunchtime for a dose, and fewer doses means fewer problems with the rebound effects of the these drugs, seen sometimes as the medication is wearing off. At these times, children may be cranky or even more active.

Treating Preschoolers

Impairment from ADHD usually begins before age six, which has led to an 180 percent increase in stimulant prescriptions for three- to five-year-olds since 1990. HMOs are encouraging quick diagnoses, working parents often can't be home to enforce structured behavior-improvement programs, and everyone seems to want a "quick fix." Yet, the eight controlled studies of forty preschoolers show variable improvement with the use of stimulants.

The challenge in treating preschoolers is to avoid treating children who appear to be "hyperactive" but don't have ADHD. It is important that a child's activity level be looked at within a developmental context: what is abnormal for a five-year-old might be normal behavior for a three-year-old. In addition, the child's symptoms must cause significant impairment and affect the child's functioning in order for a psychiatrist to consider making a diagnosis of ADHD. No one diagnostic test is available for ADHD, and the symptoms may not be specific for the condition. Symptoms that suggest ADHD very often may not become evident in the doctor's office, so a symptom history from both parents and teachers is crucial.

Psychiatric drugs may be indicated for preschoolers who show early signs of such behavioral disturbances as severe aggression or mood disturbances, where they present threats to the physical well-being of their peers, or their ability to stay in school is affected.

State legislatures are beginning to set limits on recommendations of drug use by schools in what appears to be a backlash against what some see as the overuse of stimulants. In general, these laws prohibit teachers, counselors, and other school officials from recommending psychiatric drugs for any child. These measures do not prevent school officials from recommending an evaluation by a medical doctor, but intend to make sure the first mention of drugs for a behavior or learning problem comes from a doctor. I agree that it's easier to give a child pill than to get to the bottom of the problem, and a doctor's evaluation is a must, particularly in such complex disorders as ADHD.

Drug/Class	Main Indications and Clinical Uses	Dosage (mg/kg/day or mg/d)	Select Brand Names	Adverse Effects
Stimulants				
Methylphenidate		15–60 (Ritalin); 18–54 mg/d (Concerta)	Ritalin/Methylin: 5, 10, 20 mg tab; Sustained release: 20 mg; Concerta: 18, 27, 36 mg caplet; Metadate CD 20 mg cap	Insomnia, decreased appetite, weight loss, dysphoria/Possible reduction in growth velocity during long term use/Withdrawal and rebound hyperactivity/Unmasking acceleration of mania/psychosis.
Dextroamphetamine	ADHD	10–40 mg/d	Dexedrine: 5, mg; Sustained release spansules, 5, 10, 15 mg	
Amphetamine compound		10–40 mg/d	Adderall: 5, 10, 20, 30 mg tab; Adderall XR: 10, 20, 30 mg cap	
Pemoline		37.5–112.5 mg/d	Cylert: 18.75, 37.5, 75 37.5 mg chewables	Same as other stimulants/Abnormal liver function tests and serious liver toxicity.
Antidepressants				
• *Selective Serotonin Reuptake Inhibitors (SSRIs)*				
Fluoxetine		2.5–40 mg/d	Prozac: 10 mg tab/cap 20 mg tab, oral solution 20 mg/5 ml	Irritability/Restlessness/Insomnia/Appetite decrease (acute use) or increase (chronic)/GI symptoms/Headaches/Dizziness/Flu-like symptoms during discontinuation/Complex drug interactions
Sertraline	Obsessive Compulsive Disorder/Major Depression/Other Anxiety Disorders	25–200 mg/d	Zoloft: 25, 50, 100 mg tab, oral solution 20 mg/1ml	
Paroxetine		10–30 mg/d	Paxil: 10, 20, 30, 40 mg tab, oral suspension 10 mg/5ml	
Fluvoxamine		12.5–200 mg/d	Luvox: 25, 50, 100 mg tab	
Citalopram		10–40 mg/d	Celexa: 20, 40 tab	

Antidepressants—continued

- *Tricyclic Antidepressants (TCAs)*

Drug/Class	Main Indications and Clinical Uses	Dosage (mg/kg/day or mg/d)	Select Brand Names	Adverse Effects
Imipramine	M.D.D. / Enuresis / ADHD / ADHD + Tic disorders / Anxiety disorders	2.5–5.0 mg/kg/d	Imipramine hydrochloride: 10, 25 50 mg tab Imipramine pamoate: 75, 100, 125, 150 mg cap	Anticholinergic (dry mouth, constipation, blurred vision) / Weight gain / Cardiovascular (mild blood pressure and ECG changes) / Treatment requires serum levels and ECG monitoring
Desipramine		2.5–5.0 mg/kg/d	Desipramine: 10, 25, 50, 75, 100, 150 mg tab	
Nortriptyline		2.0–3.0 mg/kg/d	Nortriptyline: 10, 25, 50, 75 mg; elixir	
Clomipramine	Same as other TCAs / OCD	2.0–3.0 mg/kg/d	Clomipramine: 25, 50, 75 tab	
• *Other*				
Bupropion	M.D.D. / ADHD	3.0–6.0 mg/kg/d	Wellbutrin: 75, 100 mg tab Wellbutrin SR: 100, 150 tab	Irritability / Insomnia / Drug-induced seizures (in doses > 6 mg/kg) / Contraindicated in bulimia
Venlafaxine	M.D.D.	1.0–3.0 mg/kg/d	Effexor: 25, 37.5, 50, 75, 100 mg tab Effexor XR: 37.5, 75, 150 mg cap	Similar to selective serotonin reuptake inhibitors / Nausea, sleepiness, dizziness, hypertension
Trazodone	Insomnia	25–200 mg/d	Trazodone: 50, 100, 150, 300 mg tab	Nausea, dry mouth, dizziness, constipation / Low blood pressure / Sedation / Priapism

Drug/Class	Main Indications and Clinical Uses	Dosage (mg/kg/day or mg/d)	Select Brand Names	Adverse Effects
Antidepressants—continued				
Nefazodone	M.D.D./M.D.D./Anxiety	50–300 mg/d	Serzone: 50, 100, 150, 200, 250 mg tab	Same as trazodone
Seligiline	ADHD in TS	5–10 mg/d	Eldepryl: 5 mg	Hypertensive crisis may occur at higher doses with dietary (tyramine) transgression or with certain drugs/Nausea/Dizziness/Changes in blood pressure
Mood Stabilizers				
Lithium	Bipolar disorder, manic Prophylaxis of bipolar disorder M.D.D. Aggressive behavior/Conduct disorder/Adjunct treatment in refractory M.D.D.	10–30 mg/kg/d, dose adjusted to serum levels in the range of 0.6–1.1 mEq/l	Lithium carbonate:150, 300, 600 mg cap/Sustained release forms: Lithobid 300 mg tab, Eskalith 450 mg tab/Lithium citrate elixir: 8 mEq (300 mg)/5ml	Frequent urination, excessive drinking, balance problems, tremor, ataxia, nausea, diarrhea, weight gain, drowsiness, acne, hair loss/Possible effects on thyroid and renal functioning with long-term administration/Children prone to dehydration are at higher risk for acute lithium toxicity—Lithium levels > 2 mEq/L can be life-threatening
Divalproex	Bipolar disorder/Aggressive behavior/Conduct disorder/Seizure disorders	15–60 mg/kg/d, dose adjusted to serum levels in the range of 50–125 mcg/l	Depakene (valproic acid): 250 mg; elixir Depakote (divalproex): 125, 250, 500 mg t; sprinkles: 125 mg cap	Sedation, nausea, liver toxicity (requires baseline and close monitoring), low platelets, pancreatitis
Carbamazepine	Bipolar disorder/Complex partial seizures	10–20 mg/kg/d, dose adjusted to serum levels in the range of 4–14 mcg/l	100 mg chewable tab; 200 mg/Elixir: 100 mg/5ml	Bone marrow suppression (requires baseline and close monitoring of blood counts)/Dizziness, drowsiness, rashes, nausea/Liver toxicity, especially under ten years of age
Gabapentin	Bipolar disorder/Seizure disorders	100–1000+ mg/d	Neurontin: 100, 300, 400, 600, 300 mg cap	Sedation, balance problems at high doses/No drug interactions

Drug/Class	Main Indications and Clinical Uses	Dosage (mg/kg/day or mg/d)	Select Brand Names	Adverse Effects
Mood Stabilizers—continued				
Lamotrigine	Bipolar disorders / Seizure disorders	75–300 mg/d	Lamictal: 25, 100, 150, 200 mg tab / Chewable: 5, 25 mg, tab	Potentially life-threatening rash
Topiramate		50–400 mg/d	Topamax: 25, 100, 200 mg tab	Cognitive difficulties (dulling, word retrieval, attention) / Dizziness, sedation
Antipsychotics				
• *Atypical Antipsychotics*				
Risperidone	Psychosis: positive and negative symptoms / TS / Augmentation in OCD / Bipolar disorder / Autism and PDDs / Aggression and agitation	0.25–4 mg/d	Risperdal: 0.25, 0.5, 1, 2, 3, 4 mg t / Elixir: 1mg/ml	Sedation / Appetite increase / Weight gain / Low incidence of muscular side effects
Olanzapine		2.5–10 mg/d	Zyprexa: 2.5, 5, 7.5, 10 mg tab	
Quetiapine		100–600 mg/d	Seroquel: 25, 100, 200 mg tab	Same as above / Concerns over potential for cataract formation
Ziprasidone		40–160 mg/d	Geodon 20, 40 cap	Less likely to cause weight gain
Clozapine	Treatment-refractory psychosis	50–400 mg/d	Clozaril: 25, 100 mg tab	Low incidence of muscular side effects / Low risk for tardive dyskinesia / Low white blood cell count (treatment requires constant monitoring of blood count) / Higher risk of seizures (dose related)

Antipsychotics—continued

• *Typical (Traditional) Antipsychotics*

Phenothiazines: Low Potency

Drug/Class	Main Indications and Clinical Uses	Dosage (mg/kg/day or mg/d)	Select Brand Names	Adverse Effects
Chlorpromazine	Psychosis/Mania/Aggressive behavior/Agitation/Self-injurious behavior/Autism	25–400 mg/d	Chlorpromazine: 10, 25, 50, 100, 200 mg tab; elixir; suppositories; injectable	Anticholinergic (dry mouth, constipation, blurred vision)/low blood pressure/Weight gain/Muscular reactions (dystonia, rigidity, tremor, restlessness, spasms)/Drowsiness/Risk for tardive dyskinesia with long-term administration/Low blood pressure especially when administered by injection/QTc interval prolongation on EKG
Thioridazine			Thioridazine: 10, 15, 25, 50, 100, 150, 200 mg tab; elixir	

Phenothiazines: Medium and High Potency

Drug/Class	Main Indications and Clinical Uses	Dosage (mg/kg/day or mg/d)	Select Brand Names	Adverse Effects
Perphenazine	Psychosis/Mania/Aggressive behavior/Agitation/Self-injurious behavior/Autism	4.0–32.0 mg/d	Perphenazine: 2, 4, 8, 16 mg tab; elixir, injectable	Anticholinergic (dry mouth, constipation, blurred vision)/low blood pressure/Weight gain/Muscular reactions (dystonia, rigidity, tremor, restlessness, spasms)/Drowsiness/Risk for tardive dyskinesia with long-term administration/Low blood pressure especially when administered by injection
Fluphenazine		0.5–10 mg/d	Fluphenazine: 1, 2.5, 5, 10 mg; elixir, injectable, long acting	

Antipsychotics—continued

- *Typical (Traditional) Antipsychotics—continued*

Other Traditional Antipsychotics

Drug/Class	Main Indications and Clinical Uses	Dosage (mg/kg/day or mg/d)	Select Brand Names	Adverse Effects
Haloperidol—high potency (butyrophenone)		0.5–10 mg/d	Haloperidol: 0.5, 1, 2.5, 10, 20 mg tab; elixir, injectable, long acting	Anticholinergic (dry mouth, constipation, blurred vision) low blood pressure / Weight gain / Muscular reactions (dystonia, rigidity, tremor, restlessness, spasms) / Drowsiness / Risk for tardive dyskinesia with long-term administration / Low blood pressure especially when administered by injection
Thiothixene—medium potency (thioxanthene)	Psychosis / Mania / Aggressive behavior / Agitation / Self-injurious behavior / Autism	1–20 mg/d	Thiothixene: 1, 2, 5, 10, 20 mg tab; elixir, injectable	
Molindone—medium potency (indole derivative)		5–150 mg/d	Molindone: 5, 10, 25, 50, 100 mg tab; elixir	Lowest weight gain among traditional agents
Pimozide—high potency	Same as other anti-psychotics / Tourette's disorder	1–4 mg/d	Orap: 1, 2 mg tab	Cardiac arrhythmias / Seizures / Muscular reactions / Drowsiness / Tardive dyskinesia

Antianxiety Drugs

- *High Potency Benzodiazepines*

Drug/Class	Main Indications and Clinical Uses	Dosage (mg/kg/day or mg/d)	Select Brand Names	Adverse Effects
Clonazepam (long-acting)	Anxiety disorders / Adjunct in treatment refractory psychosis / Adjunct in mania / Severe agitation / Severe insomnia / M.D.D. + anxiety akathisia	0.25–3 mg/d	Klonopin: 0.5, 1, 2 mg tab	Drowsiness, loss of inhibitions, agitation, confusion / Depression / Withdrawal reactions / Potential risk for abuse and dependence / Less risk for rebound and withdrawal reactions

Drug/Class	Main Indications and Clinical Uses	Dosage (mg/kg/day or mg/d)	Select Brand Names	Adverse Effects
Antianxiety Drugs—continued				
• **High Potency Benzodiazepines—continued**				
Alprazolam (short-acting)	Same as Clonazepam	0.25–4 mg/d	Xanax: 0.25, 0.5, 1, 2 mg tab	Same as other benzodiazepines / Higher risk for rebound and withdrawal reactions
Lorazepam (short-acting)		0.5–6 mg/d	Ativan: 0.5, 1, 2 mg tab injectable	
• **Atypical Anxiolytic**				
Buspirone	Anxiety disorders / Adjunct treatment refractory OCD	15–60 mg/d	BuSpar: 5, 10, 15, 30 mg tab	Drowsiness, loss of inhibitions
Noradrenergic Agents				
• **Alpha Agonists**				
Clonidine	Tourette's disorder / ADHD Aggression / Self-abuse, severe agitation / Anxiety disorders / Adjunct in mania and schizophrenia / Withdrawal symptoms	0.025–0.4 mg/d	Clonidine: 0.1, 0.2, 0.3 mg tab Transdermal patch: Catapres TTS 1, 2, 3 (delivering 0.1, 0.2, 0.3 mg/d/wk)	Sedation (very frequent) / low blood pressure (rare) / Dry mouth / Irritability / Depression / Rebound hypertension / Localized irritation with transdermal preparation
Guanfacine	Tourette's disorder / ADHD	0.5–4 mg/d	Tenex: 1, 2 mg tab	Same as clonidine: Less sedation, hypotension

Noradrenergic Agents—continued

• *Beta Blockers*

Drug/Class	Main Indications and Clinical Uses	Dosage (mg/kg/day or mg/d)	Select Brand Names	Adverse Effects
Propranolol	Akathisia/Aggression/Self-abuse/Severe agitation/Alternative to neuroleptics, especially in developmentally delayed individuals	2.0–8.0 mg/kg/d	Propranolol: 10, 20, 40, 60, 80 mg tab Long-acting 60, 80, 120, 160 mg tab	Similar to clonidine/Higher risk for slowed heartrate and low blood pressure (dose dependent) and rebound hypertension/Bronchospasm (contraindicated in asthmatics)/Rebound hypertension on abrupt withdrawal (contraindicated in diabetics)
Nadolol		20–200 mg/d	Nadolol: 20, 40, 80, 120, 160 mg tab	

• *Antihistamine, Anticholinergic*

Diphenhydramine	Sleep disorders/Agitation, acute muscular spasms	12.5–100 mg/d	Diphenhydramine: 25, 50 mg tab; elixir, injectable	Sedation, cognitive impairment, anticholinergic (dry mouth, constipation, blurred vision)/Delirium (rare)
Benztropine	Extrapyramidal reactions (spasms, muscular rigidity, tremor, restlessness)	.05–3 mg/d	Benztropine: 0.5, 1, 1 mg; elixir, injectable	

Anti-Enuretic

Desmopressin (DDAVP)	Enuresis	10–40 mcg/2	DDAVP: 0.1, 0.2 mg tab; Nasal spray: 10 mcg/spray	Headache/Nausea/Low sodium level and water intoxication at toxic doses

*Adapted from Scahill, L., Martin, A. "Pediatric Psychopharmacology II: General Principles, Specific Drug Treatments, and Clinical Practice." *Child and Adolescent Psychiatry: A Comprehensive Textbook, Third Edition* (Melvin Lewis, ed.). New York: Lippincott Williams & Wilkins 2002: 952–956.

Key

MDD = Major Depressive Disorder	TCA = Tricyclic antidepressant	OCD = Obsessive-compulsive disorder	mg/kg/d = milligrams per kilogram (child's weight)/per day
TS = Tourette's syndrome	PDD = Pervasive developmental disorder	ECG = Electrocardiogram	

Antidepressants

Depression in children often goes hand in hand with poor school performance and other problems. It may be seen in eating disorders, headaches, sleep problems, and other physical problems affecting children and teens. There are several major classes of antidepressants:

Selective serotonin reuptake inhibitors (SSRIs) are the newest type of antidepressants. Examples of SSRIs include: fluoxetine (Prozac), sertraline (Zoloft), paroxetine (Paxil), fluvoxamine (Luvox), and citalopram (Celexa). Landmark, double-blind, placebo-controlled studies of Prozac by University of Texas psychiatrist G. Emslie and Paxil by Brown University psychiatrist M. Keller show they appear to be safe and effective for the treatment of severe and persistent depression in children and adolescents. Prozac led to a 56 percent improvement in symptoms compared to a placebo, and Paxil showed a 66 percent improvement compared to a placebo. Zoloft has significantly improved symptoms among depressed adolescents in a nonblinded study, and Zoloft and Luvox have to been shown to be effective in OCD. Expert opinion doesn't support the use of SSRIs in ADHD.

Several nonblinded studies in adults with venlafaxine (Effexor), a drug that increases the levels of *both* serotonin and norepinephrine in the brain and is used to treat depression and generalized anxiety disorder, show the drug may be effective, but further investigation is necessary to see whether it really is effective.

If children have other psychiatric conditions along with their ADHD (as is true two-thirds of the time), then this must be taken into account when prescribing medication. In a double-blind, placebo-controlled trial, Prozac was effective for selective mutism when assessed by the children's parents. But teacher and clinician ratings didn't show improvements. Prozac also reduces binging in bulimia.

Tricyclic antidepressants (TCAs) are an older type of antidepressant that, in the past, were prescribed to treat depression in children, but studies do not support their effectiveness in children and adolescents for treating depression. imipramine (Tofranil) is used to treat bed-wetting in school-age children. Clomipramine (Anafranil) is used to treat OCD. Nortriptyline (Pamelor) and imipramine (Tofranil) are also prescribed for ADHD, particularly if a child is prone to tics.

Monoamine oxidase inhibitors (MAOIs) can help treat depressive disorders that also feature anxiety, but are not recommended for use in children. The major limitations associated with the use of MAOIs are significant dietary restrictions, including most cheeses, tomato sauces, and other foods popular with children, and interactions with over-the-counter medications such as cold treatments and diet pills. If the inappropriate food or medication is combined with MAOI's, a severe, potentially life-threatening medical emergency called a "hypertensive crisis" can occur. Examples of MAOIs include: phenelzine (Nardil) and tranylcypromine (Parnate).

Other atypical antidepressants that may be used in adults include: bupropion (Wellbutrin), nefazodone (Serzone), trazodone (Desyrel), and mirtazapine (Remeron). In nonblinded studies, Serzone has induced improvement in symptoms of depressed children and Wellbutrin has also improved depression among adolescent children. A black-box warning was recently added to Serzone, due to a rare but serious complication of liver failure. In addition, Wellbutrin has been studied in children with ADHD, and seems to be an effective second-line drug for children who cannot tolerate, or who do not respond to, stimulants; Wellbutrin cannot be used if there is any history of a seizure disorder, and cannot be used in patients with eating disorders.

Many ongoing double-blind, placebo-controlled drug trials are underway to examine the effects in depressed children and adolescents. The drugs under investigation include citalopram, fluoxetine, mirtazapine, nefazadone, paroxetine, sertraline, and venlafaxine.

Antianxiety Medications

Anxiety is the most common mental health problem that occurs in children and adolescents. The mainstay of treatment is cognitive behavioral therapy, but children with anxiety disorders may be treated with SSRIs. When a child faces an anxious time, such as a surgical procedure, a group of antianxiety medications that include Valium and similar drugs called "benzodiazepines" may help in the days or hours beforehand.

Several types of medications are used to treat anxiety in children: benzodiazepines, which include alprazolam (Xanax), lorazepam (Ativan), diazepam (Valium), and clonazepam (Klonopin); antihistamines such as diphenhydramine (Benadryl), and hydroxizine (Vistaril); and other medications such as buspirone (BuSpar). Antidepressants, primarily SSRIs, are also used to treat anxiety in children.

Older studies tried using alprazolam (Xanax), clonazepam (Klonopin), and imipramine (Tofranil) for school refusal. More recently, a small double-blind study using Klonopin for children with anxiety disorders showed no significant difference. Good studies with benzodiazepines have found the drugs are not effective for typical anxiety disorders, but may be for situational anxiety, for example, if a child is about to have surgery, which is the only time that I use them. I also use Klonopin for panic attacks in conjunction with an SSRI because it works fast, while it may take a few weeks for an SSRI to become fully effective. Then the Klonopin can be discontinued.

There is limited data on BuSpar in anxiety, with no controlled trials showing it is effective. There is no data on the use of Ambien in children.

Antipsychotics

Antipsychotic medications are used to treat childhood psychotic disorders, behavioral dyscontrol (including acute agitation, aggression and self-injury) seen in developmentally impaired children, perseverative behavior (such as the ritualistic behaviors seen in autistic children), depression with psychotic features, and pediatric-onset bipolar disorder.

It is important to differentiate between psychosis that is part of schizophrenia, as opposed to psychosis that is part of some other syndrome, such as a mood disorder. This is because schizophrenia overall has a worse prognosis, and also because the treatment of a mood disorder (depression or mania) with psychotic features would be different in some ways than the treatment of schizophrenia, according to research by child psychiatrist at the National Institute of Mental Health, led by R. Nicholson.

Psychotic Disorders

Haloperidol (Haldol) and chlorpromazine (Thorazine) are examples of typical antipsychotic drugs. Newer atypical antipsychotics now being studied include clozapine (Clozaril), risperidone (Risperdal), quetiapine (Seroquel), olanzapine (Zyprexa), and ziprasidone (Geodon), and several others are in the works. Some antipsychotics are also being studied to treat bipolar disorder and Tourette's syndrome. Antipsychotics have been used to treat Tourette's syndrome, including haloperidol (Haldol), pimozide, and risperidone, and the newer agent ziprasidone (Geodon). Placebo-controlled studies are in progress with risperidone.

The newer atypical agents have fewer side effects, in general, and are better tolerated, but there have been reports of problems with weight gain, seen less with Seroquel and Geodon. Clozapine, in particular, needs monitoring of blood levels each week to follow the white blood cell count. It is also important to follow the electrocardiogram (EKG), since antipsychotic drugs can sometimes lengthen the time it takes a beat to be conducted through the heart, which can predispose a child to life-threatening arrhythmias. Prolongation of the "QT" interval within the heart beat may lead to the most dangerous type of arrhythmia, and is most pronounced with the drug thioridazine (Mellaril). The QT interval can be easily measured on a routine EKG.

There are placebo-controlled studies with neuroleptic drug therapy for tics showing that pimozide and risperidone are effective.

I try not to use antipsychotics to treat tics, and make every effort not to use them chronically because of potentially serious side effects, including tardive dyskinesia and neuroleptic malignant syndrome, which may make a child acutely sick with high fever, muscle rigidity, an unstable blood pressure and heart rate, and possible kidney failure. On the other hand, severe tics can affect a child's concentration, school performance, social functioning (teasing can occur), and may even cause pain. The long-term effects are something definitely to worry about, particularly since a recent study by neuroscientist L. Burd from the University of North Dakota School of Medicine and Health Sciences showed that, when followed over the long-term, 44 percent of thirty-nine patients with Tourette's were essentially symptom free at follow-up, and only 22 percent were on medication as adults. Another study by J. Leckman from the Yale University School of Medicine found that tics begin, on average, between age five and six, and tend to get progressively worse until about age ten. From that point, tics almost always get better, and by age eighteen nearly half of all patients have no tics. Tics tend to naturally go through periods that may last weeks, where they are worse, followed by periods where they are better. For this reason, it is easy to be fooled into believing that a given medication has helped, or worsened, the tics.

Some data are available for the use of antipsychotics for mental retardation. However, the research is questionable and difficult to interpret. I will use antipsychotics occasionally in a severely aggressive mentally challenged patient who has not responded to trials of several other medications, such as mood stabilizers or beta blockers. One nonblinded study of risperidone shows it is effective, but more research is needed for me to use it.

Developmental Disorders

There are some limited data on the use of haloperidol and risperidone in developmental disorders, but much more research is necessary before they come into common usage. Recent open trials using risperidone in this population indicates some promise for the treatment of behavioral disturbance and ritualistic behaviors, according to research by A. Zuddas from the University of Cagliari, Italy.

Pediatric-Onset Bipolar Disorder

A diagnosis of childhood bipolar disorder is often met with skepticism by doctors and parents alike. This reluctance to label a child as manic has led to an underidentification of this disorder, yet a substantial number of children referred to psychiatrists can be identified as manic using a systematic assessment. In contrast to the controversy surrounding the diagnosis of juvenile mania, juvenile depression is an accepted diagnosis, and is estimated to affect at least 5 percent of children. Compared to teens with depression, those with mania show significant functional impairment, large amounts of anxiety and disruptive behavior disorders, and an increase in suicide attempts. Their moods are irritable, chronic, and often "mixed," with features of both depression and mania, according to Harvard researchers Janet Wozniak and Joseph Biederman. This is what I see clinically as well.

Unlike adults with mania, manic children are more likely to be severely irritable, with emotional storms or prolonged outbursts of mixed depressive and manic emotions. The symptoms of ADHD and mania often overlap, and are difficult to disentangle.

Drug therapy for juvenile mania should first begin with treatment of the mania, and then treatment of depression. Lastly, any anxiety or ADHD should be treated. Combinations of drugs are often necessary to take care of all of these symptoms. Small, nonblinded studies suggest that olanzapine may have antimanic or mood-stabilizing effects in acutely manic children with manic-depression and that risperidone may be effective in the treatment of juvenile mania.

Mood Stabilizers

Mood stabilizers including lithium (lithium carbonate, Eskalith), divalproex sodium (Depakote), and carbamazepam (Tegretol) may be prescribed to treat childhood mania, and have been shown in open trials to all be effective, according to research by R. Kowatch from the University of Texas Southwestern Medical Center at Dallas. Lithium is approved for manic episodes for children twelve and older, while Tegretol is not approved for use in psychiatric disorders in children. Tegretol is approved for bipolar disorder in adults, but there have been no placebo-controlled, double-blind Tegretol studies in children. Nevertheless, Depakote, lithium, and Tegretol are all used to treat pediatric bipolar disorder. Lithium seems most effective for "classic" mania (predominantly euphoria) while Depakote is more useful in "mixed" states (mania and depression comingling) or rapid cycling (many episodes of mania and/or depression that occur over the course of hours, days or weeks). Newer medication such as lamotrigene (Lamictal) and oxcarbazepine (Trileptal) seem to be effective in bipolar adults, but have not been studied children. Gabapentin has not shown to have good antimanic properties.

One lithium study of adolescents with bipolar disorder shows a 46 percent response compared to only 8 percent for the placebo group. But this study is small and had a short, six-week duration. What's clear from a study looking at the discontinuation of lithium is that children who were treated with lithium, then rapidly taken off the drug, had an increased risk of relapse. I recommend that children stay on lithium for twelve to eighteen months before considering a gradual tapering of the drug over a period of months, while watching closely for the return of bipolar symptoms.

While Depakote is widely used in children, and it is thought to be effective, there are no double-blind studies to document that, though there are open trials suggesting that it is effective, and that is what I find in my practice. I think that, in general, Depakote is better tolerated than lithium.

The main problem with lithium in adolescents is that it causes acne and weight gain. Depakote also causes weight gain, but no acne. Significant medical monitoring is required to measure the blood levels of both of these drugs. In addition, female adolescents taking Depakote should be monitored for early signs of menstrual irregularity or hirsutism (excessive hair growth on the body) since this drug may predispose women to poly-cystic ovarian syndrome (PCO). Carbamazepine tends not to cause acne or weight gain, but can be associated with bone marrow suppression, and complete blood counts must be taken regularly and followed closely.

There are many types of bipolar disorder, and different mood stabi-lizers may be more effective for these different types. Adolescents with classic manic-depression seem to do well on lithium, while those with mixed mania seem to do better on Depakote.

The guideline is a child with mixed presentation or rapid cycling would likely benefit from Depakote. Lithium is used for uncomplicated mania or pre-adolescents with very aggressive behavior problems such as conduct disorder. Also, the pattern of the illness is important. An illness that starts with depression is more likely to respond to lithium than one that starts with mania, which is probably best treated with Depakote. Other factors that predict a poor lithium response include a severe onset of the illness and delusions.

Depakote is often very effective for controlling mania and preventing recurrences of manic and depressive episodes in adults. However, because there is very limited data on the safety and efficacy of most mood stabilizers in youth, treatment of children and adolescents is based mainly on experience with adults. In addition, studies are investigating var-ious forms of psychotherapy, including cognitive-behavioral therapy, to complement medication in young people. Depakote has been shown in a small series to improve explosive temper outbursts and moodswings in adolescents, according to research by S. Donovan from the New York State Psychiatric Institute.

Other Medications

Other medications may also be used to treat a variety of symptoms. Cloni-dine (Catapres), primarily a high blood pressure medication, has become more prominent because of its wide range of indications. In addition to being used to treat severe impulsiveness in some children with ADHD and sleep disturbances, clonidine can be used to treat Tourette's syndrome and other tic disorders. Recently, there has been some concern over potential cardiac side effects from clonidine, such as low blood pressure and slowing of the heart rate. Electrocardiograms should be done both before starting clonidine and once the patient is stabilized on the drug. A child's blood pressure and heart rate should be checked periodically. Guanfacine (Tenex) also appears to have beneficial effects on hyperactive behaviors, attention abilities, tic disorders, and for "flashbacks" in children with post-traumatic stress syndrome. Compared to clonidine, guanfacine appears to be less sedating, and tends to last longer than clonidine, allowing fewer doses during the day. Recent studies have suggested that guanfacine may be effective for patients with ADHD and Tourettes, both for their tics and their ADHD symptoms.

Atomoxetine is a novel unapproved nonstimulant selective noradrenergic enhancer that has shown some success in clinical trials in treating children with ADHD who have failed to respond to psychostimulant treatment, who have the ADHD inattentive subtype, and among girls with ADHD.

Off-Label Use

It's legal for physicians to prescribe medications in ways not specifically approved by the FDA, such as prescribing psychotropic medications for children younger than age five. Prescriptions for "off-label" uses of any medication should be made only after a comprehensive evaluation has been made, and other forms of therapy, or combinations of medications that are "on-label," and therapy, have been considered, along with your child's and your personal preferences.

Whenever possible, choose a medication that is FDA-approved for children. If your doctor suggests a drug that does not have FDA approval for children, ask whether there is safety data for this drug in children or adolescents in another disorder. For example, Depakote is not approved for bipolar disorder in children, but it is approved for children with seizure disorders. That means that studies have shown the drug has a safety record, at least for some children. But that doesn't necessarily mean that your child won't develop side effects in an off-label use.

Neurology studies at the University of California at Los Angeles show that Depakote given to adolescent girls with epilepsy leads them to develop a higher incidence of polycystic ovarian disease (PCOD), a disease of the ovaries that may lead to infertility. You shouldn't automatically assume, however, that adolescent girls treated with Depakote for depression would have the same risk. The risk factors that lead to PCOD may be related to the epilepsy or to obesity, which is common in this disease. Just because side effects appear in one population doesn't mean they will occur in another population.

Lastly, if there are no data on a specific drug in children, ask whether data are available in adults. Take a very critical view of these types of prescriptions. TCAs have been proven in multiple controlled studies to be effective for adults with depression. Yet, despite many studies, they have never been proven effective for children or adolescents with depression. Children's brains are simply not adult brains. In the absence of other data, and if a child requires medication, at least have something on which to base a rationale recommendation. For instance, tricyclic antidepressants are useful for children for who have the problem of bed-wetting.

Action Plan

Any child put on medication deserves a consultation with a child psychiatrist. Child psychiatrists are best trained to do an overall assessment, which is largely based on taking a history of both the child and the family, observing the child, and conducting a comprehensive review of the domains we have discussed before, as well as the child's mental status. A full evaluation usually requires the collection of information from a variety of outside sources, such as the school, child's pediatrician, psychological testing, and social service agencies. As you can see, a child psychiatrist's evaluation is more complicated than getting a simple blood test or even a standard pediatric checkup. It usually requires several hours. The specialist looks at the current problem with attention to developmental, behavioral, emotional, cognitive, educational, biomedical, family, peer, and social components. That's why I emphasize that every child deserves a psychiatric evaluation before being put on medication for a psychiatric disorder or illness. In many cases, a child will have more than one such disorder or illness, which makes it even more important to get a full psychiatric evaluation.

A lot of factors influence each medication prescribed, including the choice of the type of medication within a given class of drugs, FDA approval, safety in another population of children, and effectiveness in adults, as I have discussed in this chapter. Lastly, you may be able to choose a drug based on what doctors call the drug's side effects profile. For example, if your doctor is going to prescribe an SSRI, you should know that fluoxetine or sertraline may cause your child to be more active than paroxetine and fluvoxamine.

If your child is using a drug that has been clinically shown to be effective in a placebo-controlled, double-blind study that should be the first approach, which would mean using fluoxetine or paroxetine in pediatric depression, for example. Then, looking at the side effect profile is a good guideline. For example, if a child is clinically depressed and is often tired and lethargic, using fluoxetine might be the better choice. If your child is anxious and has a sleep disturbance, you might choose a medication that can more easily be given at bedtime, such as fluvoxamine.

Virtually every medicine has potential side effects. But remember the side effects for not treating are the continuation of the symptoms, and the impact on the child's life and development. Many parents worry about the side effects of stimulants for their children with ADHD. But I believe that the symptoms of the disorder—profound social problems and rejection, potential impairments in self-esteem, and, in the most severe cases, academic failure or at least not achieving up to capabilities—far outweigh the risks of drug side effects in some cases. The same can be said about depression, which, if left untreated, can lead to impaired social and academic functioning, and, in the extreme, to increased risks of suicide. University of Pittsburgh psychiatrist M. Kovacs has found that the large majority of children diagnosed with a mild form of depression (dysthymia) failed to recover two years later.

The general rule for prescribing medications for children is to start low and go slow. Your child might not be at the most effective dose immediately, but the dosage can be changed as you monitor the child's progress. The most common response child psychiatrists hear is that the medication doesn't work. An appropriately prescribed medication taken at a sufficient dose over a sufficient amount of time is most likely to elicit a response. So give it a chance to do what it's supposed to do.

You also need to know that your child's response to different medications will likely occur within different time frames. Some drugs, such as psychostimulants, work almost right away. You should see some effects within one to two hours, depending on the medication prescribed. For antianxiety drugs, a response may take a few days to a few weeks, depending on the medication, to two months. With antidepressants, you may not see a response for up to two months. Make sure to ask the important question: "When will we expect to see a response from the medication?"

Don't be confused if your doctor prescribes an antidepressant for some other condition, such as bed-wetting, anxiety, or pain. As I've noted, in adults SSRIs help irritable bowel syndrome even when the patient is not depressed. As a close colleague of mine, Boris Rubinstein has said, "the medicines don't know that they are antidepressants." A medication called one thing may be useful for another symptom.

"Evidence-based medicine" is a term that's often thrown around in evaluating the appropriateness of a medication. The gold standard for a research study is a double-blind, placebo-controlled, randomized trial. In this special kind of study neither the researcher who is evaluating the treatment nor the patient who is receiving it knows which patients are receiving the treatment. Other types of less objective medical studies may report results that are biased. The researchers may have a biased assessment of the patients' response, based on how they want the patients to react. Or the patients may develop a placebo response, hoping that just by taking a treatment, any treatment, they will feel better. Therefore, you need to ask your doctor not only whether there has been research on a drug, but also the type of research, specifically, was a double-blind, placebo-controlled trial conducted.

When you see a consultant, in a sense you are hiring him or her to do the background research on your child's condition and treatment, and to digest it for you. But you can search the medical literature yourself using MEDLINE through the PubMed Web site (*www.ncbi.nlm.nih.gov*) to find research on specific drugs. Many landmark studies in child psychiatry are also referenced by the NIMH and American Academy on Child and Adolescent Psychiatry Web sites. Multiple studies have shown the effectiveness of psychostimulants—probably the most studied medications in child psychiatry—on ADHD. Lots of books and booklets for the public, as well as specific disease Web sites, are available. You'll find them referenced in the back of this book.

Action Points

1. Get a psychiatric evaluation before putting your child on drug therapy for a psychiatric disorder or illness.
2. Besides the class of drug, base your choice of medication on whether the drug: is FDA approved; safe and effective for your child's condition (or another similar condition); is effective in adults; and has acceptable side effects.
3. Since the drug dosage may be low at first, give it time to work.
4. Know how soon to expect a response to the drug.
5. Ask your doctor whether there have been double-blind, placebo-controlled studies of the drug for your child's condition.
6. Do research on any prescribed drugs through medical text books and the Internet.

CHAPTER 17

From Heating Pads to Hypnosis— Easing Pain and Anxiety

*E*very parent can become an expert at distraction using hypnotic techniques to relieve pain and anxiety. Most of these strikingly simple techniques can be used easily by children or taught to them by their parents. The best distractions capture attention through sight, sound, and touch, which is based on the pain theory that a child (or adult, for that matter) can't pay attention to two different things at once. If a child's attention is focused elsewhere, the painful impulses may pass by without notice.

One of the hardest things for parents is divining the cause of anxiety or pain. This often is tied up in the child's expectations. Sometimes asking, "What are you afraid of?" instead of simple reassurance does the trick. Often, children can't verbalize it, and that's the time to use distraction techniques.

Some interventions work for some ages, but not others. This chapter includes a chart listing age-appropriate techniques for reducing pain and anxiety in children, adapted from work by British Columbia Children's Hospital psychologist Leora Kuttner, Ph.D. The methods incorporate physical, behavioral, and imagination-based distractions.

Preschoolers

Penny, a shy four-year-old, is terrified because she needs to have an intravenous line put into her wrist. I ask her to imagine that a "magic glove"

I will put on her hand will numb the pain of the needle. Slowly and ceremoniously I put the invisible glove on her hand, one finger at a time, recounting a story of how the glove is magic and will protect her from pain. Once the glove is "on," I test by using a light pin-prick on each hand. Penny clearly states that she feels the pin-prick less on the hand with the magic glove. After several practice sessions with her mother's help, we put on the magic glove, and her IV line is inserted with minimal discomfort. This technique was borrowed from a tape put out by the Canadian Cancer Society called "No More Tears."

Translation: "I'm frightened because the needle will hurt, and it might go right through my hand. Maybe the magic glove is not 'real,' but it works!"

Young children are extremely suggestible. Often, rapid rocking, patting, and stroking is all it takes to calm down an anxious infant. Allowing the child to suck on a pacifier or bottle, humming to her, playing music,

Helpful Strategies for Children to Reduce Pain and Anxiety

Age Level	Physical	Behavioral	Imaginative
Preschool (ages 2–5)	Rocking Presence of parent Ice/heat Stroking Patting	Party blower Blowing bubbles Pop-up books Viewmaster Music Favorite stuffed animal or blanket Glitter wand Hidden-picture books Singing	Storytelling Speaking to the child through doll or stuffed animal Favorite stories or favorite places Story tapes
School-age (ages 6–11)	Relaxation technique Raggedy Anne or Andy Ice/heat Stroking Blowing breath out	Music Video games Number games Hidden-picture books Bubble blowing	Favorite place or favorite activity Riding a bike Playing in playground
Adolescence (ages 12–18)	Relaxation technique Heat/ice Blowing out breath	Music with headphones Video games	Self-hypnosis Sports activity Favorite place Driving a car

or visually stimulating her with mobiles that change shape and color also work well.

For toddlers, a temperature change tends to soothe acute injuries, for example, putting ice on a bumped head or a heating pad on a tummy-ache. A party blower helps establish slow, rhythmic breathing. Blowing bubbles, pop-up books, a View Master, music, and a favorite stuffed animal or blanket help distract the preschooler. Telling a story or speaking to the child through a doll or stuffed animal helps the child become actively involved. You can also use the "magic glove" pain-reduction technique described in the anecdote, or obtain a videotape of the technique from the Canadian Cancer Society.

Happy Land Game

I have created a game for preschoolers and young school-age kids to help them with anger, anxiety, depression, and day-to-day activities, such as getting them up, dressed, and out of the house in the morning. The game teaches how to get from place to place—Sleepy Land, Mad Land, Worried Land, Happy Land, School Land, among others—using behavioral and cognitive techniques. For example, to go from Worried Land to Happy Land takes four spaces—on space number 1 you breathe deeply and relax your muscles; on space number 2, you use "self-talk" ("I know monsters aren't real."); on space number 3, you use imagery (Make believe you're floating on a cloud.) Space number 4 is Happy Land. Parents can individualize the game by looking at their child's symptoms (Is it anger? Fear of robbers?) and their interests—for example, imagine you're as powerful as a Pokémon character, or swooshing through the snow carving perfect turns. To get from Sleepy Land to School Land, the child follows certain steps—gets dressed, eats breakfast, brushes his teeth, puts on his backpack—and receives bonus points for getting to the next step before a timer goes off. The game also provides fun tips—for example, create a wire model of the child and dress it together the night before from head to toe.

School-Age Children

Owen, a rough-and-tumble six-year-old, can take a basketball hitting his face without wincing, but screams at the sight of a needle to have blood drawn. Unfortunately, due to a mild blood disorder, he needs to have monthly blood tests. The problem seems to be getting worse, taking three nurses to hold him down, so he was referred to me.

I show Owen a breathing exercise using a party blower, with his mother coaching him. "This reminds me of my husband coaching me through labor," she remembers. After two office visits and several practice sessions at home, we do a dry run using all of the props, except the actual needle. This goes quite smoothly and earns Owen several stickers and some ice cream. The following day, he confidently gears up for the actual blood-draw, humorously ordering the nurses out of the room. He holds his own arm still as he breathes in and out through the party blower while his blood is taken. This technique was borrowed from friend and colleague Ken Gorfinkle, Ph.D., a specialist in using nonmedical treatments for pain.

Translation: "I hate having my blood drawn because it hurts. Being held down makes me feel out of control."

Distractions work for the school-age child as well. By just being there, along with stroking, patting, and ice or heat when appropriate, a parent may ease pain and anxiety. Another physical technique is to make like Raggedy Anne or Andy, Gumby, or a wet noodle, that is, having the child imagine having no muscle tone. Muscle relaxation is known to reduce anxiety and pain. Here's a simple method school-age children can learn: Count to three as you breath in, hold for one second, then breathe out while you count to six in your mind. Repeat several times.

You can build up the types of behavioral techniques for school-age children to include singing together, telling favorite stories, and imagining, and then, in the child's mind, going to a favorite place or doing a favorite activity. Hidden-picture books help shift the child's focus away from what makes him hurt or nervous. The more sensory modalities the child uses, the better the distraction technique. That's why computerized video games are so useful for distraction, because they stimulate through vision, sound, and touch all at once.

I also use colors. Most children associate one color, usually red, with pain. I instruct them to imagine a soothing color of their own choice. School-age children can be taught to draw a picture of the mind as the control center and to turn off the pain switch in their heads before going through an anxious or painful event.

Bubble blowing is fun and exciting to do. I had clowns blow bubbles in the cardiac catheterization lab to relieve anxiety during procedures with children, and it worked well. But the cardiologists were afraid that the soap might get into the equipment and contaminate the sterile field. The clowns were able to find other creative distraction techniques to soothe the children having their hearts catheterized.

Cognitive and behavioral approaches can also help overcome fear. A model developed by Temple University psychologist Philip Kendall can change the way kids think. It is called "Coping Cat," and it instructs them on how to note their feelings and expectations, then to act upon them and adapt their attitudes, leading to rewards and positive responses by their parents. "Coping Cat" uses a workbook with weekly homework that is reinforced with visits to the therapist. Children just have to remember the acronym "FEAR." The program asks children to first realize that they are feeling frightened (F). Then they see that they are "expecting bad things to happen" (E) and try to figure out what scary thoughts are behind the frightening feeling. Then they pick some "activities and attitudes" (A) that will help them through the experience. Finally, they see the responses and choose rewards (R) to help them feel proud.

The Terrible Teens

Ron, a brash fifteen-year-old, was born with a congenital heart condition that requires him to have yearly catheterizations of his heart. He never seemed to get used to the high-tech setting of the catheterization lab, with all the monitors, fancy equipment, and doctors gowned "like aliens." I suggest that he use his portable stereo cassette player during the next procedure. With the din of heavy metal music barely audible to the doctors and nurses, Ron tolerates the procedure quite well, and comments that he "got lost" in the music.

Translation: "This place weirds me out and makes me feel jumpy. Having to be here makes me feel different. And I'm PO'd that my friends are down at the shore and I'm stuck here."

The main issues for teens are control over discomfort and how to capture their attention. More options are available to relieve anxiety and pain, including listening to music with headphones and self-hypnosis using a favorite sport, place, or activity, such as driving a car. Teens can easily learn to use the step-by-step self-hypnosis program outlined in Chapter 15.

Action Plan

Behavioral interventions such as deep breathing, muscle relaxation, guided imagery, and hypnosis are quite effective for both pain and anxiety. Many research studies show these techniques work well for pain, including research by my Columbia colleague Ken Gorfinkle, M.D. He has trained children with cancer, whose treatment requires taking repeated blood samples, to use a party blower while the blood is being drawn. With parents coaching them during the process, they reported much less distress. The most dramatic example comes from Herb Spiegel who trained an obstetrician to deliver a baby cesarean section rather than using hypnosis anesthesia.

Getting a child out of a particular unpleasant psychological state, even briefly, can have carry-over effects. If a child is anxious, and you distract him, even after the distraction stops, he will still feel less anxious.

With younger children, you have to use more games and age-appropriate symbols—a cartoon character may help put the magic glove on the child's hand. Refer to the list of Anxiety/Pain Reduction Techniques to come up with a distraction that's appropriate for your child's age. For example, when my nine-year-old daughter Hannah was stung by a bee, I put ice on it and watched a television show with her while we waited for her pain to subside. Once the ice had melted and the show had ended, she felt less distressed and more comfortable from a combination of the ice easing the pain and having me sit with her. Basically, these techniques help you take common sense to another level. You can use distraction and reassurance in just about any situation where your child is uncomfortable or frightened.

If distraction doesn't work when your child is frightened, try refocusing or cognitive restructuring. This means that you look at what your child fears and discuss whether those fears are realistic. Appeal to the child's rational side. Recruit intelligence and intellect, not emotions. Ask such questions as, Is this likely to happen? Is it a realistic thought? What can you do when you think that? How do you know this will happen? What makes you so sure? How else might you react? What else can you say to yourself to ease the fear? What else might you do?

To a certain degree, preparation will help. At the eleventh hour, distraction might work just as well. Perhaps your child is nervous about playing in a big baseball game or a test or going away from home. For the big game, if your child is nervous because she's the starting pitcher, remind her she's been practicing for weeks, and that she knows to step off the mound and take a deep breath if she's nervous. The night before the game, you might go out to movie, read a book together, listen to music, or do something to take her mind off the game. Use a combination of things, and be flexible. If she's worried, talk about her feelings. You might tell her to just do her best, and even if the team loses, there will be lots of other games. Remind her about the Olympic swimmers who listen to music through headphones before they swim to relax and to psych themselves up.

All children should develop ways to deal with anxiety all of the time. So use these situations to practice anxiety and pain-reducing techniques.

Action Points

1. Use age-appropriate distraction techniques to help ease your child's pain or anxiety.
2. Try refocusing your child's attention by discussing the situation in a rational way.
3. Have your child practice these techniques so he or she can use them when needed.

CHAPTER 18

Sugar and Spice and St. John's Wort— Alternative Medicine

*B*rian, an extremely moody sixteen-year-old, was having bad migraine headaches. He was constantly getting into fights with his friends, and claiming that they were provoking him. In addition, Brian had become overweight-he ate too much junk food, refused to exercise, and wouldn't join any sports teams. He began a real battle with his parents. I met with Brian in conjunction with his neurologist, and we decided to treat his migraines with valproic acid.

For his moodiness, I recommended fish oil, which has been found to be an effective mood stabilizer in adults with manic depression. I also referred him to a weight loss center specializing in adolescent obesity, where Brian would attend group therapy, meet with a dietitian, and exercise. Three months later, Brian had lost 15 pounds, he was less moody, and his headaches had nearly vanished. His parents became less angry with him once they realized that Brian wasn't being lazy and not helping himself.

Translation: "I feel like a failure because I can't lose weight on my own, so why bother trying anymore."

In the twenty-first century, physicians will have to use alternative interventions or they will lose their patients. Both the public and health researchers have become savvy to the positive effects of alternative remedies. More than one-third of Americans now use at least one alternative therapy, and the number of visits to alternative medicine practitioners in the United States is increasing rapidly. In the oncology department at Columbia University, one survey by Kara Kelly showed that 84 percent of parents report using alternative remedies for their children, and about half of them did not tell their doctors about it. Some 75 percent of the parents felt that the alternative remedies were helping (although their doctors did not always agree with this). This points out the importance of being able to feel that you are doing something for your child and not just watching what the doctors do.

Whether it's essential oils for eczema, herbs for otitis media, or vitamin C for stress, parents are using alternative therapies. Families of children with asthma and allergies often seek so-called alternative treatment as supplementation, not as a real alternative to traditional medicines (complementary instead of alternative treatment). Atopic dermatitis treatments comprise a mixture of acupuncture, homeopathy, and dietary regimens.

This chapter provides a critical review of alternative medicine, including natural products and nutritional supplements as potential treatments for childhood diseases.

Children Use CAMs
(Complimentary and Alternative Medicine)

Surveys show that CAM therapies are frequently used to treat children, mostly by parents who also use CAM therapies. Also, a large proportion of children who are taking herbal supplements are also taking prescription or over-the-counter medications at the same time.

University of Pittsburgh researchers surveyed the use of CAM among children visiting an emergency department. A review of 525 completed surveys identified sixty-three parents (12 percent) who acknowledged that they had used at least one form of CAM therapy to treat any of their children.

Homeopathic and naturopathic remedies were the most common therapies used. Parents most often used CAM therapies to treat respiratory problems, and were most influenced by word-of-mouth. Children who were treated with CAM therapies were more likely to have a parent who also used such therapies. Twelve (40 percent) of thirty families who reported using either an herbal or homeopathic remedy also used a prescription or over-the-counter medication at the same time to treat their child. About 70 percent reported informing their child's physician of their use of CAM therapies.

More than 20 percent of parents who receive traditional health care have also used CAMs for their children, according to research at the Children's National Medical Center in Washington, D.C. There was no difference in the use of CAMs based upon the child's ethnic background or parent's socioeconomic status. The most common types of alternative medicines used were vitamins, nutritional supplements, and herbal remedies. The most common reasons for using them were frequent respiratory infections, asthma, headaches, and nose bleeds.

In contrast to the Pittsburgh study, the majority of parents who used alternative medicines did not tell their pediatricians about it. While most vitamins and nutritional supplements will not react negatively with traditional medicines, some herbal remedies can cause serious reactions.

Pediatricians Speak Out about CAM

CAM has become ingrained in our society. In its first policy statement on the subject, the American Academy of Pediatricians asked its members in mid-2001 to get more involved in counseling parents about alternative medicine. The group said doctors should become more aware of the vitamins, teas, herbs, and procedures used outside mainstream medicine and should help parents evaluate the pros and cons of a particular therapy.

Although the Academy focused its recommendation on parents of children with developmental disabilities and chronic disease, the policy extends to parents of healthy children. The organization acknowledged that up to one-third of Americans have used alternative medicine in recent years and up to 50 percent of children with autism in the United States may have been given some alternative medicine.

Parents are using vitamin supplements and other unproven treatments to treat children with autism. The unconventional treatments include the nutritional supplement dimethylglycine, a mixture of vitamin B_6 and magnesium. In some cases, parents are getting prescriptions for antifungal medications for their autistic children in the belief that a fungus may be responsible for the disorder.

Many parents of children with chronic illness and disability are choosing CAMs, and quite often pediatricians aren't even aware of this. The goal of the Academy's guidelines is to encourage practicing pediatricians to continue to provide a scientific perspective as well as information on treatment options. Among their recommendations, the association is advising doctors to seek outside information and share it with families; evaluate the scientific merits of specific approaches; identify risks; avoid dismissal of alternative medicine in ways that communicate a lack of sensitivity and concern; guard against becoming defensive; and assist in monitoring a therapy if a family decides to use an alternative medicine.

The Feds Study CAMs

Even the federal government is studying alternative medicines. In 1998, the National Institute of Health (NIH) established a research center to study pediatric CAM at the University of Arizona in Tucson. The NIH is currently researching the use of echinacea and osteopathic manipulation to prevent ear infections; guided imagery and chamomile tea to help children with abdominal pain; and acupuncture and osteopathic manipulation to ease muscle tension in children with cerebral palsy.

As I've indicated, hypnosis and similar techniques can help children cope with pain. Ongoing studies of relaxation, guided imagery, and self-hypnosis are being conducted by pediatricians at the University of Arizona to help children in controlling and easing asthma symptoms and for recurrent abdominal pain.

Happiness with Herbs

Sean, an unruly eighteen-year-old with a penchant to verbally abuse his mother, is about as sullen as a young adolescent can get. His family is in turmoil. Sean's grades are dropping due to concentration problems, and the battles at home have escalated due to his rampant irritable, oppositional behavior. Sean refuses to take antidepressants, but he agrees to try St. John's Wort because it is a naturally occurring herb.

"Within three weeks of taking the St. John's Wort, his mood turned around 180 degrees," says his mother. "He has become pleasant, agreeable, and even takes out the garbage without a fight." With newfound optimism, Sean turns back to his studies, and his grades improve significantly over the next semester.

Translation: "I'm moody because I'm frustrated over my schoolwork and about disappointing my parents, and their anger at me just makes it worse. I'm not taking any medicine because that would mean I'm 'psycho.'"

Herbs, supplements, and other naturally occurring substances are being used to treat many types of childhood psychiatric problems and mood disorders. St. John's Wort is used for mild depression; alpha omega fatty acids, including fish oil, for mood instability; and inositol (a natural chemical that resembles glucose) for obsessive-compulsive disorder and panic disorder. Other herbal remedies have been used in conditions from autism to migraines. I also use glycine and alpha omega fatty acids for schizophrenic adolescents.

St. John's Wort

One of the best known uses of herbs is St. John's Wort for mood elevation. Several controlled studies have shown positive results in treating adult patients with mild to moderate depression, with improvement in such symptoms as sadness, helplessness, hopelessness, anxiety, headache, and exhaustion with no reported major side effects. The herb's action is based on the ability of the active ingredient, hypericin, to inhibit the breakdown of chemical messengers in the brain. The herb works as a serotonin reuptake inhibitor, which means it acts in ways similar to drugs prescribed for depression. In fact, in Germany, nearly half of depression, anxiety, and sleep disorders are treated with hypericin.

For centuries, St. John's Wort also has been used as a putative incontinence treatment in children. Herbalists usually suggest the child drink a tea made of the herb just before bedtime.

But St. John's Wort is not risk free. It should not be taken with any other antidepressants; it is not effective for severe depression; and you should not stop taking any prescribed medications for depression without telling your doctor. It can also precipitate mania in bipolar patients. Since there is no data on using it in children or adolescents, I would be quite cautious in recommending it. While side effects are rare, they may include gastrointestinal discomfort, fatigue, dry mouth, and hypersensitivity to sunlight. The NIH has also issued an alert that St. John's Wort may interact with antiviral medications, specifically indinavir, a protease inhibitor used to treat HIV, and cyclosporine, a drug used to reduce the risk of organ transplant rejection. The National Center for Complementary and Alternative Medicine warns that the herb also reduces the effectiveness of some prescription drugs, so consult your doctor before adding it to your child's drug regimen.

Acupuncture for Various Ailments

Acupuncture has been tested in children with various physical ailments. A small Israeli study is the first to describe acupuncture as a successful treatment of constipated children. A small Swedish study shows that acupuncture may increase skin temperature in some children who have cold hands and feet due to neurological problems. Acupuncture is one of the alternative therapies being used to treat depression among adults.

No one knows exactly how acupuncture works. The 5,000-year-old Chinese explanation is that it balances the flow of vital life energy, called "*qi*" or "*chi.*" According to the Chinese, qi can become imbalanced by heat, cold, dampness, emotions, diet, exercise, and the spirit. Acupuncture rebalances the flow of qi by inserting special needles at 360 points along energy pathways, or meridians. A more Western explanation is that acupuncture works by triggering the release of endorphins, one of the body's natural painkillers. Acupuncture is now practiced by more than 10,000 licensed acupuncturists, who treat more than 1 million Americans each year.

CAM Studies in Children

New research reviewed below indicates that a variety of CAM therapies are being tested for children with headache pain.

Biofeedback for Headache

An alternative treatment for children suffering from tension headaches may be a biofeedback technique that shows children how to warm their hands. In a small study from North Dakota, five children, ages eight to fourteen, were taught the hand-warming technique over six sessions. The results confirm that children who learned the hand-warming skill, and practiced it on a regular basis during treatment, learned how to better manage their pain. All of the children had clinically significant reductions in frequency, duration, or intensity of their headaches following biofeedback. Six months after learning the technique, four of five children were headache free.

CAM for Pain

A wide variety of CAM therapies are being used for childhood pain in more than 70 percent of university-affiliated pediatric pain management programs, according to a study at Children's Hospital in Boston. Some fifty-two pediatric pain management programs were identified, and forty-three (83 percent) responded to a telephone survey directed to a physician or nurse from the pain service program. More than 70 percent said they use CAM therapies. The services offered include biofeedback (at 63 percent of the centers); imagery (60 percent); relaxation therapy (60 percent); massage (49 percent); hypnosis (44 percent); meditation (44 percent); acupuncture (40 percent); art therapy (28 percent); music therapy (23 percent); self-help groups (19 percent); therapeutic touch (14 percent); herbal remedies (9 percent); chiropractic (7 percent); yoga (5 percent); and tai chi (2 percent).

For more ways to handle pain, see Chapter 17.

Homeopathy for Reducing Stress

Homeopathy is based on the principle that very small amounts of an ingredient that cause a certain symptom in a healthy person will cure that same symptom in a sick person. The theory is that homeopathic remedies rally the body's own natural healing defense to fend off illness. Remedies are prepared using microdoses of plant, mineral, and animal substances, which are diluted and then shaken vigorously. It is a form of complementary medicine that relies heavily on observation and experience. Homeopaths prescribe medicine only after looking at all of a person's symptoms.

Homeopathic practitioners claim that their remedies can be useful in treating stress in a child. They emphasize that, like traditional medicine, it is sometimes useful to refer to a homeopathic guide or expert in order to correctly match your child's symptoms to the proper remedy. Some of the more frequently used homeopathic remedies for stress reduction found in health food stores include:

- *Kali bromatum,* which is supposed to be especially useful to alleviate fearfulness, nervousness, worry, and restlessness, particularly related to physical or emotional exhaustion.
- *Ignatia amara* to relieve sadness and tearfulness. It may be helpful after an emotionally stressful episode.
- *Agaricus muscarius* is purportedly very helpful for counteracting sullenness.
- *Tarentula* is geared to excitable and restless children.
- *Stramonium* is said to be particularly useful for an anxious and fearful child, perhaps in a reaction to a situation involving shock or fear.
- *Valeriana officinalis,* the active ingredient in valeria, may help alleviate anxiety, sleeplessness, and instability.

With homeopathy, practitioners claim that the worst that can happen is nothing. The only potential harm comes from continuing treatment with an ineffectual ingredient. But the time lost using an ineffective treatment can never be made up. As I've described, many other well-recognized stress-reducing techniques are available for children that I would highly recommend over homeopathy, or which could be done along with homeopathy. It is important for parents to research what they will be give their child and not relinquish this responsibility. I would also point out that I would not necessarily rely on faith that these treatments could not have side effects on your children. Let the user beware!

Unhealthy Health Supplements

In 1994, the U.S. Congress gave the Food and Drug Administration the responsibility to regulate the safety of dietary supplements. A broad array of herbs, amino acids, botanical extracts, vitamins, and minerals can now be marketed without FDA approval, unless they positively demonstrate a danger to people.

Some "health" supplements have proven to be unhealthy. At least six herbal remedies—kava, chaparral, comfrey, germander, lobelia, and yohimbe—can trigger serious toxic reactions. Lecithin may contain impurities, such as heavy metals and pesticides. And, although tryptophan is a naturally occurring essential amino acid, a contaminant introduced in its manufacture in 1990 led to 1,500 cases of a debilitating muscle disorder, eosinophilia myalgia syndrome. Some parents are giving children gingko to combat attention deficit disorder, but gingko isn't appropriate for children. Its blood-thinning power could cause excessive bleeding if a child gets cuts or scrapes. Seizures have also been reported in children after ingestion of large quantities of ginkgo seeds.

Since herbal medicines are readily available in the United States—not only in health food stores, but also in drug stores and even grocery stores—without prescriptions, most consumers assume they are harmless. Consequently, they use herbs to self-treat a variety of conditions, and to boost their body's overall functioning, and their children's, too. But this use of herbal medicine, which dates back to 2800 B.C.E. in China, can cause serious side effects.

Children may be even more susceptible to some of the adverse effects and toxicity of herbal products. They have a different physiology from adults, an immature metabolic system, and, in most cases, weigh less and therefore should not take the same dose as an adult. Although information promoting the use of herbal medicine is widespread, true evidence-based information about the effectiveness and safety of herbal medications is limited. Parents who provide herbal remedies to their children need to follow the results closely, in particular monitoring for adverse effects and interactions, and talking to their pediatrician before trying them.

One of the ways children are exposed, sometimes unknowingly, to herbs is through dietary supplements in drinks. Major drink manufacturers are now adding in several dietary supplements at a time into their "energy" or "tonic" drinks. These ingredients include: taurine, inositol, ginseng, guarana, kava, valerian, ginkgo, creatine, Echinacea, yerba mate, yohimbe, and St. John's Wort.

Kava and Liver Damage

Kava *(Piper methysticum)* is an herbal remedy sold as an alternative pain reliever, relaxation aid, and memory enhancer. However, reports from

Germany and Switzerland suggest that kava may damage the liver. A number of cases of liver toxicity associated with the use of kava products have been reported internationally, including one death and several patients who required liver transplantation. The British and Swiss governments have prohibited the sale of all products containing kava extract.; Canadian health officials have warned consumers not to use any products that contain kava, which may be an ingredient in herbal and homeopathic preparations sold to treat anxiety, nervousness, insomnia, pain and muscle tension.

In the United States, the National Institutes of Health have suspended two studies of kava and the Food and Drug Administration is reviewing cases of adverse events that may be linked to kava use. The FDA also sent out a letter asking doctors to review potential cases of liver toxicity that may be related to kava. Canadian officials also advise consumers to contact their physicians if they experience any adverse effects from taking products containing kava. The following symptoms may be associated with liver problems: jaundice (yellowing of the skin or whites of the eyes), brown urine, nausea or vomiting, unusual fatigue or weakness, and stomach or abdominal pain.

The kava situation and the absence of federal regulations to protect consumers remind us to read the labels on all herbal products. I also suggest doing Web research. You will find tens of thousands of references to kava on the Web. I would recommend such sites as the FDA's *www.fda.gov* and the American Botanical Council's Web site, *www.herbalgram.org*.

Potentially Dangerous Herbs for Children

The following list, taken from the Brown University *Child and Adolescent Psychopharmacology Update* March 2002 newsletter, shows which herbs can be dangerous to children and why:

- **Comfrey:** If taken internally, comfrey can impair blood flow to the liver and result in liver failure.
- **Ephedra** (also known as Ma Huang): Used to relieve bronchial congestion or asthma induced bronchial constriction, ephedra is a stimulant that can increase heart rate and blood pressure, possibly resulting in dizziness, insomnia, and vomiting.

- **Homegrown mint:** This mint is difficult to differentiate from Pennyroyal, which can result in liver failure and death.
- **Senna, cascara sagrada, buckthorn bark:** These substances can cause profound diarrhea and, over time, may result in electrolyte imbalance that can lead to heart problems.
- **Willow bark:** The salicin in willow bark may cause stomach irritation and Reye's syndrome in children.

Not All They Should Be

Another potential problem with herbal remedies is that they may not contain all that they are supposed to. The popular herbal supplement valerian, which is often used as a sleep aid, is one such product. A report from ConsumerLab, a commercial testing company that regularly examines herbal supplements, says that many valerian products have serious quality-control problems.

Of the seventeen valerian products they tested, only eight passed the lab's tests. Four contained none of the herbal source of valerian, *Valerian officinalis*, and four had only about half the amount they claimed to have. To find the results of this and other supplement tests, go the company's Web site at *www.consumerlab.com*.

Dangers of Some Chinese Herbs

The consumption of Ba-baw-san, a Chinese herbal medicine, has been significantly associated with increased levels of lead in the blood of Chinese children. The consumption of such Traditional Chinese Medicine (TCM) can have adverse health effects, especially among children. Life-threatening bradycardia with rapid onset and central nervous system and respiratory depression developed in three unrelated children in Colorado during 1993 following ingestion of Jin Bu Huan tablets, a Chinese herbal medicine used for relieving pain.

Consumer Beware

Parents who are interested in providing herbal preparations for their children should consult their pediatrician to make sure that the herb they are considering is not potentially toxic or will not cause an adverse reaction, either on its own or in combination with other pharmaceutical medications. A long list of herbs can be toxic, including the following:

Herbal Remedies and Their Toxicities

Common Name	Botanical Name	Purported Use	Toxicity
Aloe	*Aloe vera*	Wound healing, general tonic, laxative	Diarrhea, nausea/vomiting
Black cohosh	*Cimicifuga racemosa*	Premenstrual syndrome, menstrual pain, dyspepsia	Nausea/vomiting, uterine contractions
Broom	*Cystisus scoparius*	Sedative	Vomiting, uterine contractions, slow heartbeat
Burdock	*Arctium lappa L* or *Arctium minus*	Blood purifier	Diuresis, anticholinergic poisoning
Chapparal	*Larrea tridenta*	Analgesic, anti-inflammatory, diuretic, expectorant	Liver toxicity
Comfrey	*Symphytum officinale*	Blood purifier, stomach ulcers, wound healing	Liver toxicity
Echinacea	*Echinacea augustifolia* or *E. purpurea*	Immune system booster	Central nervous system stimulant, dermatitis, anaphylaxis
Ginseng	*Panax ginseng*	Adaptogen, aphrodisiac	High blood pressure, agitation, anxiety, depression, insomnia
Golden seal	*Hydrastis canadensis*	Upset stomach	Nausea/vomiting, central nervous system stimulant, paralysis, respiratory failure

continued on next page

Herbal Remedies and Their Toxicities—*continued*

Common Name	Botanical Name	Purported Use	Toxicity
Hawthorn	*Cratageus laevigata* or *C. Monogyna*	Angina	Low blood pressure
Juniper	*Juniperus communis*	Gout, diuretic, upset stomach	Kidney toxicity, seizures, hallucinations
Kava kava	*Piper methysticum*	Sedative	Dermatitis, hallucinations, shortness of breath
Licorice	*Glycyrrhiza glabra*	Diuretic	Low potassium levels, high blood pressure, edema
Lobelia	*Lobelia inflata*	Stimulant	Nausea/vomiting, seizures, headaches
Ma huang	*Ephedra sinica*	Stimulant, asthma	Mania/psychosis, high blood pressure, fast heart beat
Passion flower	*Passiflora caerulea*	Sedative	Seizures, low blood pressure, hallucinations
Pau d'Arco	*Tabebuia impetiginosa* or *T. avellanedae*	Blood purifier, cancer cure	Nausea/vomiting, anemia, anticoagulation
Poke root	*Phytolacca americana*	Arthritis	Liver toxicity
Sassafras	*Sassafras albidum*	General tonic, stimulant, antispasmodic	Liver toxicity, liver cancer
Valerian	*Valeriana officinalis*	Sedative	Possible dystonic reactions and liver toxicity
Yohime bark	*Pausinystalia yohimbe* or *Corynanthe yohimbe*	Aphrodisiac, stimulant	Hallucinations, anxiety, high blood pressure, fast heart beat, nausea/vomiting

Source: *Psychosomatics*, Vol. 39, No. 1, p. 8, January–February 1998.

When buying herbs, look for ingredients with the U.S.P. (U.S. Pharmacopoeia) notation, which indicates manufacturers have followed their standards. Many pediatricians are open to using herbal remedies to supplement traditional health care, for example, suggesting echinacea to ward off cold symptoms. For more information about herbal medications, visit the FDA Web site at *www.fda.gov.*

When dealing with herbs, follow these general guidelines:

- Talk to your pediatrician about the herbs you want to use. You may also want to consult a qualified herbalist.
- Read the labels carefully. Try to get products that do not combine herbs, particularly if you mean to take only one.
- Don't take an herb for longer than the manufacturer's recommendations.
- Make sure the label says the herbal product contains a standardized extract, meaning that it has a known level of the active ingredients.
- Watch out for allergic reactions. If you suspect your child is having a reaction—hives, itchiness, even difficulty breathing—call a doctor immediately.
- If you can, find out whether the company producing the herb is reputable, and whether quality-control standards have been met.

Watch What You Mix

Some parents "get into" alternative medicine because their friends take it, or because they began searching the Web for more information. Others may be frustrated with the standard medications handed out by their pediatrician. Still others are convinced that using herbal remedies for minor ailments that the common cold goes along with weekly chiropractic and massage sessions.

But most parents remain wary, and for good reason. Most of the information surrounding CAM therapies is purely anecdotal, virtually none of it is evidence-based, and very little has been tested on children.

It's easy to get carried away and think just because a CAM remedy is portrayed as natural that it is safe. Simple lifestyle changes, such as a good diet and regular exercise, are often more important for children's health than acupuncture and herbal remedies.

There are potentially dangerous interactions between herbal medicines and prescription drugs. St. John's Wort acts as an antidepressant and should not be added to prescription antidepressants; bromelain, a pineapple extract, can interact with anticoagulants; eucalyptus oil induces liver enzymes and can increase the metabolism of certain drugs, while sassafras does just the opposite; and licorice can act as a diuretic and should not be used along with prescription diuretics. Here's a list of some of the potential interactions of herbs with drugs:

Potential Drug Interactions of Herbs

Herb	Potential Interaction
Bromelain	Enhances the activity of coumarin anticoagulants.
Buchu, Boldo, Uva ursi	Diuretic activity can increase the effectiveness and the toxicity of heart glycosides by potassium loss.
Chapparal, Comfrey, Groundsel, Gordolobo (Pyrrolizidine-containing herbs)	Concurrent use with medications that induce liver enzymes, such as dilantin and phenobarbital, leads to increased liver toxicity.
Cinnamon	Retards the breakdown of tetracycline and methylcycline.
Eucalyptus oil	Induces liver enzymes into action. Reduces half-life of metabolized drugs.
Hops, Kava kava, Passion flower, Valerian	Sedative activity can add to that of alcohol.
Jimson weed, Lobelia, Thornapple, Burdock root	Anticholinergic activity can add to that of medications with anticholinergic properties.
Ink cap	Contains disulfuram. Produces an antabuse-like reaction when taken with alcohol.
Licorice	Concurrent use with diuretics can lead to low blood potassium. May counteract antihypertensive action of some prescribed medications.
Mellilot, Tonka beans, Woodruff	Contains natural coumarins.
Sassafras	Inhibits liver enzymes. Increases the half-life of metabolized drugs.

Source: *Psychosomatics*, Vol. 39, No. 1, p. 9, January–February 1998.

Action Plan

The main issue I have with herbal remedies is that they are pharmacologically active, just like all medications. I look at herbs as another form of drug treatment. Anytime a child needs more than one medicine, I introduce them one at a time to watch for the effects, whether good or bad. If the child had a reaction to a group of medicines all introduced at once it would be difficult to determine which was causing the reaction.

Don't be deceived by the "natural" label. Yes, they may be natural, but that doesn't mean that herbs are safe. Herbal supplements are now being added into beverages, so be aware of what your children are drinking. Check with your doctor if your child is on medication before taking herbs. Remember that herbs interact with other herbs and drugs, and that herbs can have side effects. If you really want to give your child herbal medicines, include your doctor in your decision to help you monitor any interactions.

You can keep a log that tracks the symptoms you're trying to treat using the Monthly Mood Chart in Chapter 1, ranking each symptom on a scale of 0 to 3. It's best to get a baseline of symptoms before you intervene with an alternative therapy. You can be fooled by the natural fluctuations in your child's moods, or by placebo effect—the expectation that you or your child has that the herb will make them feel better. A few weeks of the log will give you a sense of this natural ebb and flow. After the baseline period, use the alternative medicine for two to four weeks, then review your child's response to the remedy with your doctor.

There's a lot of misinformation about herbs and other wild stuff out there. I recently reviewed the Library of Medicine database and found 7,000 references just on herbs. Be particularly wary of information about an alternative product written by the company that produces or sells it. If you go to an Internet chat room, remember to take what you get there with a grain of salt. Word of mouth is not very reliable. Word of mouth or media hype often has misled people into thinking an alternative therapy was a "wonder cure." Parents of autistic children were all excited when CBS's *60 Minutes* ran a television feature about the incredible successes with secretin treatments.

Unfortunately, the limited research that has been done to date does not back up these claims, though it is being studied further.

Go to established sources of information about alternative therapies. In response to the widespread use of botanical therapies in America, the Medical Economics Company has published a new *Physicians' Desk Reference for Herbal Medicines*. This book provides details on more than 600 herbal medications, which are not subject to the same safety and effectiveness testing required by prescription drugs. It includes the scientific and common names of herbs along with information on when to use them, when not to use them, dosages, and literature citations. To order, call 888-859-8053.

Obtaining information about vitamins, minerals, and selected herbal and botanical agents has become a great deal easier through the use of the Internet. The Office of Dietary Supplements at the NIH has a database of bibliographic information on the Web at *http://ods.od.nih.gov/databases-databases.html*. You can search three different databases using more than 1,000 key words to identify scientific information on dietary supplements.

Other sources of information on herbs and supplements include the Federal Trade Commission (*www.ftc.gov*), National Center of Complementary and Alternative Medicine (*www.nccam.nih.gov*), Quackwatch Medical Fraud Homepage (*www.quackwatch.com*), the National Medicines Comprehensive Database (*www.naturaldatabase.com*, which requires a subscription), and the National Center for Homeopathy (*www.homeopathic.org*).

Use skepticism when evaluating citations of references you receive from the Internet. Look at the methods of the study. Ask yourself a few questions: How many subjects were in the study? How good is it? Is it relevant? There may be sufficient information included in the abstract to evaluate a study's usefulness, but in general you really have to go to the original article to make your best determination about the study's value.

My take, in general, on alternate medicine is to be careful to evaluate the side effects and discomfort associated with treatments. I've heard of children with allergies who have had extensive testing by alternative practitioners that included many injections of immunological substances of questionable effectiveness. When considering whether to use an alternative medicine, determine how much discomfort it might cause your child, how invasive it might be, the potential side effects, and how well established it is. I'm more likely to recommend an alternative medicine, such as certain vitamins or herbal therapies, if they don't cause pain or side effects. In that regard, I follow the basic medical precept, first do no harm.

Once in a while, I'm pleasantly surprising about something I read or hear about from a colleague about alternative treatments. But many things children can take are good for them. In general, I believe that children should take a daily multivitamin, as my children do. It's best to help your child eat a balanced meal and get vitamins from natural sources. But a multivitamin is good protection in case your child doesn't eat well from time to time. And remember, nothing substitutes for a balanced diet.

I get a little concerned about giving SAM-e to depressed children since the current data show its effects only for adults. Developing brains are influenced differently by medications. Just because a substance is safe for adults, and helps them feel better, it doesn't necessarily mean it's safe for children.

Action Points

1. Herbs are like medicine, which means they have actions and interactions. Enlist your doctor's help and knowledge when using them.
2. Track your child's reaction to alternative remedies using the Monthly Mood Chart.
3. Trust established sources for information about remedies more than hearsay, particularly on the Internet.
4. Provide your child with a daily multivitamin to ensure good health.
5. Children are not simply small adults, and may react differently to alternative therapies than adults.

CHAPTER 19

Child 2001—
Wellness in the Next Millennium

*T*oday's children's lives are unlike those of their parents. Our children's world is one:

That has always included MTV, remote controls, and powerful
  computers
That has always included AIDS
In which half of them live with only one parent
In which half of them are overweight
In which more die from accidents than from disease
That has been irrevocably changed as a result of the World Trade
  Center attack and ongoing threats of terrorism.

Each child has unique needs, strengths, and weaknesses. In this chapter, I offer guidelines for parents, in particular, how to reestablish their roles as parents. I'm calling for a move away from total immersion in work and a return to the family as the anchor of the next generation. Parents who learn more about child development and how to understand their children will be the most successful.

Looking Out for Your Children

Potential threats to children's health include violence, obesity, drug abuse, sexually transmitted diseases (STDs) such as HIV, the growing computer culture, information overload due to media saturation, terrorism, and the dissolution of the American family.

Violence

Parents can learn how to evaluate their concerns about aggressive behavior by looking at their own behavior toward children and others and at the influence of violence in the media. The causes of violence, including school violence, are complex, and there are no magical solutions. But, schools, communities, and parents can take steps to help keep children safe.

Children as young as preschoolers can become violent. While parents may hope the child grows out of it, violent behavior in a child at any age should always be taken seriously. The range of violent behavior among children and adolescents may include explosive temper tantrums, physical aggression, fighting, threats or attempts to hurt others (including homicidal thoughts), use of weapons, cruelty toward animals, fire setting, intentional destruction of property, and vandalism. We need to pay more attention to teens, especially when they start showing signs of depression, or get into trouble with the law. These signs need to be taken seriously.

A complex interaction or combination of factors may increase the risks of violent behavior among children and teens, according to the American Academy of Child and Adolescent Psychiatry (AACAP). These factors include: previous aggressive or violent behavior; being the victim of physical abuse and/or sexual abuse; exposure to violence in the home and/or community; a family history of violence; exposure to violence in the media; use of drugs and/or alcohol; presence of firearms in the home; a combination of stressful family factors such as poverty, severe deprivation, the breakup of a marriage, single parenting, unemployment, and loss of support from extended family; and brain damage from a head injury.

Violent children are often the victims of violence themselves. Common emotional experiences of violent children include experiencing aloneness, abuse, and separation from their family. These children may feel more isolated after a critical event in their childhood in which they did not have the support of a caring adult.

Children who have several risk factors and display certain violent behaviors should be carefully evaluated by a mental health professional.

These behaviors include intense anger; frequent loss of temper; extreme irritability; extreme impulsiveness; and becoming easily frustrated. Early professional treatment can often help the child to learn how to control anger or express anger and frustrations in appropriate ways, and to be responsible for his or her actions and to accept the consequences. Treatment may also address family conflicts, school problems, and community issues.

Reducing or eliminating these risk factors goes a long way in preventing violence. Parents can also decrease the exposure of their children to violence in the home, community, and through the media. Research shows that violence begets violence.

Preventing Violence in Our Schools

Vermont psychiatrist David Fassler, M.D., co-author of *Help Me, I'm Sad*, has developed a common sense ten-point plan that addresses school violence that I endorse. His ten points are:

1. Identify kids with problems.
2. Reduce class sizes.
3. Reduce access to guns.
4. Promote tolerance and teach conflict resolution.
5. Eliminate bullying.
6. Provide access to mental health care.
7. Improve awareness and communication.
8. Develop peer support programs.
9. Expand access to drug and alcohol treatment.
10. Enhance parent and community involvement.

By working together, parents, teachers, and communities can develop effective strategies to identify kids who need help, and intervene as early as possible. According to Dr. Fassler, such an approach would ultimately lead to safer schools and a better educational experience for our children.

In one of the first studies ever to compare existing school-based aggression prevention programs across the nation, researchers from the Children's Hospital of Philadelphia found that targeting programs to kindergarten and young elementary school students, focusing on aggression in girls as well as boys, and conducting programs in naturalistic settings such as playgrounds are key factors in the success of aggression prevention in schools.

We often think of school violence as fist fighting between high schools boys, but in reality, aggressive behaviors begin to express themselves at a very young age. And while violence is more common among boys, it appears among girls as well, but is expressed in different ways. By defining aggression broadly to include both physical aggression and relational aggression—gossiping, threatening to exclude from the peer group—effective aggression prevention programs may be better able to target both boys and girls and focus on the everyday acts of aggression that occur on school playgrounds that can lead to more serious violence in later years.

While extreme acts of violence, such as school shootings, get the media attention, more often it's the verbal threats, name-calling, and insults that can be heard in school hallways. One way to deal with these behaviors is through conflict resolution training. Such training can increase students' knowledge of nonviolent means to resolve conflict, facilitate a more positive attitude about nonviolent conflict resolution methods, and reduce the frequency of violent confrontations in school.

Gun Violence

Parents do a reasonably good job of making their homes safe for children—except when it comes to locking guns away where children can't get at them. Most parents practice injury prevention, including having their children wear seat belts in cars and helmets on bicycles, maintaining functioning smoke detectors and fire extinguishers at home, and keeping electrical outlets covered, and water heaters not turned up too hot. But many gun owners don't store their guns unloaded and fail to store them in a locked compartment.

Accidents aren't the only reason to keep children safe from guns. Nationally, among young people ages ten to eighteen, more than half of gun deaths are homicides, and more than one-third of gun deaths are suicides. Most teens who commit suicide do it with a gun they find in the home. If it is difficult to get hold of a firearm because it is locked up, unloaded, and the ammunition locked and stored separately, suicidal teens will have a cooling off period before they can hurt themselves.

While school shootings such as those as Columbine and Santana are rare, the presence of guns in schools is not. Between 8 percent and 10 percent of U.S. high school students carry guns to school every day, according to *School Violence: Assessment, Management, Prevention,* edited by Mohammad Shafii, M.D., and Sharon Lee Shafii, R.N., B.S.N. In a typical midsized city, thirty to fifty cases of school violence are reported daily, and half of these cases involve guns, the book reports.

Most children involved in extreme school violence exhibit signs of problems well beforehand. We need to identify them as early as possible and make sure they get help. We also need to teach children to let a responsible adult know when other children threaten gun violence. Children should not have to make the decision whether another child is really serious or not about using a gun.

How to Talk about War and Terrorism

In an age when pictures are transmitted instantaneously, there is no way to shield children from disturbing news. Although we can see an event before we can understand what happened, parents are not powerless to control how the news affects their children. It is important to make sure that parents take the time to talk with children about such events as war and terrorism—with the TV off. Parents need to listen to their children's worries and answer questions about their fears, and to their children what rumors they have heard. Spending time together in this time of crisis will pay off later when children have more personal crises.

When explaining the details of war to a young child, parents should reassure them. Emphasize that the major reason we went to war was so that we can be safe from harm and continue to do things without being afraid. If children are worried they did something wrong, it's critical to reinforce that they did nothing to cause the war.

Parents should also look for symptoms that indicate their children are being affected by the war talk and images. Younger children, when stressed, often become more anxious; sometimes they can become aggressive and defiant, refusing to go to bed or hitting friends and siblings. Older children may have angry outbursts and experience physical symptoms, such as headaches or stomach pain. Other grieving-type behavior may include anxiously clinging to an adult for comfort, or a wish

to sleep with a parent for reassurance during the night, as well as conduct problems, including aggression or stealing, according to child psychiatrist Robert Pynoos, M.D.

The younger the child, the more likely it is that play will show the
emotional effects, such as violence; reenactments of the trauma; rough-
ness; shooting imaginary guns in a repetitive way, as an attempt to master
the trauma; and art productions and storytelling that may be graphic, possibly bloody, with lots of color and emotion.

It's okay for children to want to focus on something else besides the
war. If they are more interested in cartoons, the pennant race, or the latest
new movie, all the better. Let them live their lives. Parents should provide
structure and support for the activities of daily life with minimal disruptions.

Upon hearing about terrorist attacks, children may worry about what
the future holds. Parents need to field as many questions and concerns
as they can. Children may be afraid of bombs, nuclear attacks, biological
warfare, and chemical warfare. We need to reassure them that our governments are doing a lot to prepare for these threats by increased security in our country and all over the world. And we need to show them
what measures we are taking to ensure that our homes are safe, including
locks, alarms, and safety bars.

Some children who are already coping with loss and fear will need
special reassurance. These include children who have parents away from
home, who are involved in a divorce, who are hospitalized, who have lost
a loved one recently, or who are especially worried about safety, stability,
and security. Parents with these at-risk children must make special efforts
to offer physical, emotional, and intellectual nurturing and support.

Obesity

According to the Centers for Disease Control and Prevention, 14 percent of six- to eleven-year-old children and 11 percent of twelve- to seven-
teen-year-olds are overweight, which means that more than 5 million
American children are overweight. That number has been steadily
increasing since the 1960s, when nearly 5 percent of both children and
adolescents were overweight.

Obesity is an easy medical condition to recognize, but difficult to
treat. Generally, a child is considered obese when his or her weight is at

least 10 percent higher than what is recommended for that height and body type. Obesity most commonly begins in childhood between the ages of five and six, and during adolescence. Studies have shown that a child who is obese between the ages of ten and thirteen has an 80 percent chance of becoming an obese adult.

Obesity has a negative effect on both physical and mental health. The physical consequences include increased risk of heart disease, high blood pressure, diabetes, breathing problems, and trouble sleeping (sleep apnea). There's also an increased risk of emotional problems. Teens with weight problems tend to have much lower self-esteem and to be less popular with their peers. Depression and anxiety may also occur.

While genetics plays a major role in childhood obesity, environmental influences also have a strong effect. Television, video games, unsafe neighborhoods, and microwaves all contribute to the new national epidemic of childhood obesity. Television and videos lead to a sedentary lifestyle, while unsafe neighborhoods help keep children indoors. The average child sees 10,000 food advertisements a year, and 80 percent of commercials on children's programs are for food products. The convenient microwave oven means many children select and prepare their own meals, and children tend not to make healthy choices.

Children are also snacking on more empty calories. They are eating more salty snack foods such as potato chips, drinking more sugared beverages or soft drinks instead of milk, and not eating enough fruits and vegetables. That means the snacks are becoming a source of empty calories or junk food in the child's diet, which can contribute to obesity.

Snacking in itself isn't bad. In fact, young children need to snack because their stomachs are still very small. Parents and children need to learn how to incorporate nutritious snacks into their diets. Parents purchase most of the food eaten in the home; if parents make available only healthy food snacks, children will start to eat them.

As children get older, more of their snacking happens outside the home as they tend to stay at school longer and are involved in sports and other activities. Parents can pack something nutritious and satisfying in backpacks that children can eat on the go, such as fruit, a bagel with peanut butter, or bite-size vegetables. Many foods children love also give them some nutrients, in particular calcium, which they may be lacking, including string cheese, chocolate milk, and yogurt. Keep them handy for children's after-school snacks.

As America's children grow larger, many people might suggest that they be put on a diet or a vigorous exercise regimen. But a diet can harm children by depriving them of important nutrients. Children should not be put on a diet, unless guided by a registered dietitian or physician. Instead, I recommend a moderate, not strenuous, amount of exercise before restricting the amount of food a child eats.

The government's Dietary Guidelines for Americans, published in 2000, recommends that children engage in one hour of moderate physical activity most days of the week, if not daily. This means sixty minutes total, not necessarily continuously, and can include riding a bicycle, skating, dancing, jumping rope, swimming, playing tag, or taking part in physical education or sports during or after school.

The guidelines encourage parents to set good examples for their children by eating sensibly at home, playing games or participating in other physical activities with their children, and limiting their television and computer game time.

When it comes to mealtime, keep it positive, relaxed, and fun. Parents can get children involved with choosing and preparing healthy foods and snacks. They also can help children learn what it feels like to be hungry and to have a full stomach, which can help reduce eating out of boredom or habit. A regular meal schedule is important as well. Regular mealtimes can help children develop normal eating schedules, improve hunger control, and decrease overeating.

Parents should never use food as a reward or punishment. Some parents restrict the food intake of one child because he or she is overweight and allow other children in the house to eat whatever they want. Such a practice sets up the potential for an eating disorder.

The family focus should be more on improving health and less on what children weigh. Modify how everyone in the house eats and perceives food. Setting up foods as "good" or "bad" is not helpful. Everyone in the house, regardless of weight, should develop balanced eating habits.

Parents of an overweight child often become obsessed with the child's losing weight, but not all overweight children grow up to become overweight adults. If the entire family adopts a healthy lifestyle, an overweight child will be more likely to become a healthy adult.

Drug Abuse

Many teens experiment with alcohol and drugs. Unfortunately, they often don't link today's actions with tomorrow's consequences. Teens also have a tendency toward the Superman Syndrome—they feel as if they are indestructible and would never succumb to the problems associated with alcohol and drugs. But using alcohol at an earlier age increases the risk of using other drugs later on.

More than two in five American high school seniors used an illegal drug, such as marijuana, in the 2000–2001 academic year, the first time the rate has edged up in four years, according to a survey of more than 75,000 students by the National Parents' Resource Institute for Drug Education (PRIDE). While rates of illegal drug use have largely stabilized among students twelve or older, alcohol use has dropped to the lowest level in more than a dozen years. Even so, more than half of all students from grades six through twelve drank alcohol during the 2000–2001 school year, according to the survey, which is used by schools and federal policymakers to guide antidrug efforts.

Efforts to reach early teens with antidrug messages seem to have successfully reduced drug use by junior high (grades six to eight) students over the past five years. However, during that same period, use among twelfth graders remained flat. Perhaps it's time to target older students with antidrug strategies.

The PRIDE survey found teen drug use was higher (38 percent) among those who lived with their father only, compared to those living with both parents (20 percent). Among seniors, the survey found that 41.4 percent had used at least one illegal drug during the 2000–2001 school year, up from 40.2 percent the year before and about the same as the rate in the 1996–1997 school year. More than one in five took drugs once a week. The illegal drugs cited were marijuana, cocaine, uppers, downers, inhalants, hallucinogens, heroin, and steroids. Drug use among junior high school students declined marginally last year to 13.7 percent, continuing a decline from 20.7 percent five years ago.

Another national survey confirms that teen alcohol and drug use has stabilized. The National Household Survey on Drug Abuse, an annual check on drug, alcohol, and tobacco use in the United States, shows that, among children ages twelve to seventeen, 9.7 percent said they had used

an illegal drug in the past month in 2000. The rate for 1999 was 9.8 percent. Drug use was less common, however, among teens who believed
their parents would strongly disapprove if they tried marijuana once or
twice. About 7 percent of these teens reported using an illicit drug in the
previous month. Among teens who believed that their parents did not
strongly disapprove of marijuana use, 31 percent reported using drugs in
the past month. These findings, based on interviews with a nationally rep-
resentative sample of more than 71,000 people aged twelve and older,
offer hope that more and more young people are making the decision not
to do drugs. Clearly, parents have a key role in their child's decisions.
One teenager I was treating pined about the fact that her parents did not
come down hard on her for using alcohol, telling me that if they had, she
definitely would have drunk less.

The drinking rate remained about the same among teens, with about
27 percent of those ages twelve to twenty saying they had consumed
alcohol in the past month in 2000.

Parent's Alcoholism and Behavioral Problems

For several decades, a parent's alcoholism has been associated with
increased psychiatric or behavioral problems in children. Iowa researchers
led by psychiatrist Samuel Kuperman, M.D., now suggest that children of
alcohol-dependent parents are at greater risk for several different types of
childhood psychiatric disorders. When a parent has both alcoholism and
antisocial personality disorder (ASPD), the alcoholism seems to contribute more to a child's behavioral difficulties.

Probably the worst type of alcoholism involves those who drink and
who also have aggressive behavioral problems. However, the Iowa
research shows that in families with alcoholism and ASPD, the children's
psychiatric problems are related more to the parents' alcoholism than to
the ASPD. People with ASPD are prone to getting into fights, have difficulty holding down jobs or putting down roots, tend to be promiscuous,
violate general societal rules, and are at increased risk for suicide
attempts.

The Iowa study is part of an ongoing, six-site collaborative study on
the genetics of alcoholism. The researchers analyzed interviews of 463
children ages seven to seventeen and their biological parents. The results

show that parental alcoholism increases the likelihood of childhood ADHD, conduct disorder, and anxiety disorders, and the combination of parental alcoholism and ASPD puts children at greater risk for oppositional defiant disorder (ODD).

Boys tended to have more problems with the three disruptive disorders—ADHD, conduct disorder, and ODD. Girls showed more anxiety problems, such as separation anxiety. Older children tended to have more conduct disorder problems than younger children, which had been suspected in the past, but had never been demonstrated. It's likely that these children are predisposed to having some sort of problem, and that at different ages and in different genders the disorders are expressed differently.

The Iowa researchers also found that dysfunctional family interactions between the parents and the children were associated with increased risks for the development of conduct disorder, alcohol abuse, and marijuana abuse in their children. That brings up the question: If family relations can be improved, can these symptoms be improved? Further research will have to answer this provocative question.

Sexuality and STDs

One-half of sixteen-year-olds in the United States are sexually active, and many of them participate in unprotected sexual intercourse that results in sexually transmitted diseases (STDs), including infection with human immunodeficiency virus (HIV), the virus that causes AIDS.

The lethal risks associated with HIV are frightening for both parents and teens. More than 25 percent of people infected with HIV acquire the virus as teens. Sexual intercourse of any type—vaginal, anal, or oral—can transmit the disease. It's important for teens to learn the rules of safe sex, particularly the use of condoms, and to be able to talk about sex and negotiate with their sexual partner to protect themselves.

Some red flags may indicate that a teen is involved in dangerous sexual risk-taking. These include participating in unprotected intercourse, having sexual relations with an untrusted partner, feeling victimized or abused, or like he or she is abusing or victimizing someone.

Before teens become sexually active, they need to ask themselves several important questions, suggests Lynn Ponton, M.D., author of *Sex*

Lives of Teenagers: Revealing the Secret World of Adolescent Boys and Girls. These questions include whether they are engaging in sexual activity for themselves; whether they feel rushed by the situation; whether their bodies feel ready; whether they trust their partners; and whether they would be comfortable saying, "No," even at the last minute.

Parents know they should guide their child through teenage, but when they think about talking with them about sex, they often back off. Ponton suggests that parents be direct, use simple language, and admit to their own embarrassment. She says that adolescence is about taking risks, sexually and in other ways. Parents will want teens to have safe, healthy options, even if this means engaging in activity that runs counter to their own values.

Teens look to parents for advice about how to assess positive and negative risks. Parents need to help their teens learn how to evaluate risks and anticipate the consequences of their choices, as well as to develop strategies for diverting their energy into healthier activities when necessary. Parents also need to pay attention to their own risk taking. Teens are watching, and imitating, whether they acknowledge it or not.

Another place where today's teens face risky sexual encounters is through online sexual solicitation. To assess the risk factors surrounding online sexual solicitations, New Hampshire researchers conducted a telephone survey of a random sample of 1,501 children ages ten to seventeen who were regular Internet users. Nearly one in five (19 percent) of them were the targets of unwanted sexual solicitation in the last year. Girls, older teens, troubled youths, frequent Internet users, chatroom participants, and those who communicated online with strangers were at greater risk. One-quarter of the solicited youth reported high levels of distress after solicitation incidents. Those most likely to feel distressed were the younger ones, those who received aggressive solicitations (for example, the solicitor attempted or made offline contact), and those who were solicited on a computer away from their home.

Many young people who use the Internet encounter unwanted sexual overtures. Parents should be prepared to educate their children about how to respond to online sexual solicitations, including encouraging them to disclose and report such encounters, and to talk about them.

On the other hand, many teens use the Internet as a source of health information, and STDs and sexuality are two of the most explored topics.

Researchers at Mount Sinai School of Medicine in New York conducted a school-based survey of a socioeconomically and ethnically diverse sample of 412 suburban New York tenth graders to examine their Internet use and attitudes toward accessing health information through the Web. Half of the students had used the Internet to get health information, and the topics most often explored included STDs; diet, fitness, exercise; and sexual behaviors. When considering eleven separate health topics, girls found it more valuable to have information on birth control, diet and nutrition, exercise, physical abuse, sexual abuse, and dating violence. So the Internet can be a valued source of information on a range of sensitive health issues.

Computer Culture

Just as we don't fully realize the psychological consequences of high-tech medicine, our understanding of the "side effects" of information technologies lags behind. The magnetic attraction of the Internet and video games can be insidious. They can detract from physical activity because children don't go out and just play, and they interfere with real-time, real-life interpersonal relationships. Fast-paced video games and music videos limit children's abilities to pay attention to less stimulating tasks and events. Communication skills have been reduced to short sound bites.

The digital age is here to stay. It's up to parents to put technology in perspective and to communicate both its staggering potential and its inherent limits. While most parents teach their children not to talk with strangers, not to open the door if they are home alone, and not to give out information on the telephone to unknown callers, they need to provide the same kind of guidance and supervision for a child's online experience. Most chat rooms or newsgroups are completely unsupervised. With anonymous screen names, children may not know if they are "talking" with another child or a pretender.

Children may access areas of the Internet that are inappropriate or overwhelming for them. They may download information that promotes hate, violence, and pornography. Or they may be misled and bombarded with intense advertising.

To help parents choose computer resources that are age appropriate, the Entertainment Software Rating Board rates video games, interactive software, and entertainment Web sites for children. I also suggest that for increased safety, parents place the computer in a common area of the home rather than in a child's bedroom. Parents need to be involved in helping a child choose which Web sites to visit.

Violent video games may mildly increase aggressive thoughts, aggressive feelings, and arousal, which might explain why they increase aggressive behavior, according to Iowa State psychologists, who reviewed thirty-five studies conducted through 2000 on the effect of violent video games on more than 4,000 children and adults. Some parents don't think twice about letting their children play violent video games, but the effects may not be trivial. Parents need to be aware of what types of computer games their children are playing and make a rational choice based on their specific child, and use their own judgment.

Video games that reward success are an excellent motivating tool. But when the goal is to hurt or kill, you have to wonder about the message the game maker is trying to convey. Long-range studies of children after they have played these games show a reduced tendency to intervene when others become mean or violent. When they get angry, tired, or stressed, they are more likely to respond aggressively.

But even video games rated *E* for "Everyone" contain a significant amount of violence, according to Harvard researchers led by Kimberly Thompson, ScD. They created a database of all existing *E*-rated video games available for rent or sale in the United States by April 1, 2001. Then they identified the distribution of games by genre and characterized the distribution of content associated with these games. Finally, they played and assessed the content of a convenience sample of fifty-five *E*-rated video games released for major home video game consoles.

They found that about two-thirds of the games they played involved intentional violence for an average of about one-third of the game play. Injuring characters was rewarded or required for advancement in 60 percent of the games. Not surprisingly, action and shooting games led to the largest numbers of deaths from violent acts, and they found a significant correlation between the proportion of violent game play and the number of deaths per minute of play.

So even *E*-rated games, which are supposed to be analogous to *G*-rated films and suitable for all audiences, may be a source of exposure to violence for children and may reward players for violent actions.

Reduce Video, Reduce Aggression

Reducing video game playing and television watching may lessen aggressive behavior in children. A Stanford University study involved third and fourth graders from two schools. One school went through a six-month program that consisted of eighteen motivational lessons of thirty to fifty minutes each to reduce video game and television time, a ten-day recommended ban on television, and a then limit on video and television time to seven hours at most per week. The other school served as a control.

At the study's end, the children who had gone through the program had reduced their video game playing and their television viewing by about one-third. Their aggression, which was rated by their peers, was significantly lower compared to the control group's. They also had significantly lower levels of verbal aggression and playground aggression, and perception of the world as "mean and scary" was also reduced. The effects were similar in both boys and girls, and tended to be larger for children who the researchers had noted were more aggressive before going through the program.

Media Overload

Following a groundswell of public concern, as well as White House and Congressional conferences on children and violence, a coalition of health organizations over the summer of 2000 condemned media violence as harmful to children. The statement by the American Academy of Pediatrics, American Medical Association, and AACAP was based on more than 1,000 research studies over three decades that link media violence to aggressive actions, attitudes, and values.

A subsequent sweeping survey of research on media violence, sex, and risky behavior over the last ten years concurs that what children watch can directly influence their behavior. The Johns Hopkins University survey by Susan Villani, M.D., reflects the growing concern about the impact on youngsters of the sexually suggestive, violent, and aggressive content that frequently permeates the media today.

The media categories studied included television and movies, rock music and music videos, advertising, video games, and computers and the Internet. The study shows that the primary effects of media exposure are increased violent and aggressive behavior, increased high-risk behaviors, including alcohol and tobacco use, and accelerated onset of sexual activity. While newer forms of media have not been as adequately studied as television, the researchers say they are concerned with the increasing amount of time the average child spends with increasingly sophisticated media.

The classic studies linking TV violence and aggression and youth behavior were done in the 1970s and 1980s, with material that wasn't very violent by today's standards. But now, it's more violent and more graphic and more sexual. Children are being exposed to more graphic content at younger and younger ages.

Research in the past decade has strengthened previously reported links between television violence and increased aggressive behavior in preschoolers. Risky behavior depicted in entertainment media has been associated with increases in sexual activity, drinking, smoking, and drug use. Viewers of violent television content may learn aggressive behaviors and attitudes, and may become desensitized to violence and fearful of being victimized. Even children's cartoons are becoming violent, with depictions of violence having increased steadily.

Preschool children who frequently watch violent television shows or play violent video games are much more likely to engage in aggressive, destructive, and antisocial behavior, according to New York University School of Medicine researchers. Their study evaluated the influence of television programs or video games featuring realistic violence such as gun shootings, fights, explosions, and killings on the behavior of seventy-nine preschool children between the ages of two and six. The researchers used a standard measure, called the Child Behavior Checklist, and asked parents about their children's behavior, including whether they were disruptive, fought with other family members, hit other children, and destroyed property. Parents also were asked about their children's habits regarding television and computer games, including how frequently their children watched television violence and played violent video games. Frequent exposure was defined as several times a week or more.

The researchers found that children who were frequently exposed to media violence were eleven times more likely to exhibit high levels of aggressive and antisocial behavior compared with children in the study who weren't frequently exposed. This association was independent of other influences, including the child's age, dysfunctional parent-child interactions, involvement with child protection services, and witnessing domestic violence (15 percent of the families reported domestic violence).

This study's results underscore the need for parents to get more involved with their children. The American Academy of Pediatrics offers the following recommendations regarding media violence:

- Limit television-viewing time to one to two hours a day. (I would recommend less.)
- Make sure you know what television shows your children watch, which movies they see, and what kinds of video games they play.
- Talk to your children about the violence that they see on television shows, in the movies, and in video games. Help them understand the effects of such violence in real life and the serious consequences for violent behaviors.
- Discuss with your children ways to solve problems without violence.

If their child sees an inappropriate commercial on television, parents should take the time to discuss it right away. Over the past decade or so, marketers have increasingly targeted the 27 million youth that are nine to fourteen years old, the so-called "tweens" who are midway between early childhood and adolescence. Highly charged and highly sexual marketing efforts that once were reserved for adults are now being targeted to tweens. Parents can help their tweens and teens by paying attention to their purchasing, downloading, listening, and viewing patterns, and by helping them identify destructive ideas presented in the media.

American Family

Childhood was rarely the idyllic, carefree time portrayed in popular 1950s television shows such as *Father Knows Best* and *Leave It to Beaver*. Real children have always experienced growing pains. But there is a new consensus that life is more difficult for today's children. They live with new worries such as AIDS and terrorist attacks, with an increased awareness of such realities as sexual abuse and serial killers, and they often confront firsthand the breakdown of the twenty-first-century family.

One out of every two marriages today ends in divorce, leaving many children to live with one or the other parent. Children of divorce are usually frightened and confused, and feel threats to their security. Children often believe that they are the cause of the divorce, and may want to assume responsibility for bringing their parents back together. The traumatic loss of one or both parents through divorce may lead children to become more vulnerable to physical and mental illnesses. But a family's strengths can be mobilized during a divorce, and children can be helped to deal with this often difficult situation.

Parents involved in a divorce should be aware of distress signals from their child. Young children may become more aggressive, uncooperative, or withdrawn. Older children may feel deep sadness and loss, may develop behavior problems, and their schoolwork may suffer. Children of divorce often have trouble with their own relationships and experience problems with self-esteem.

Research shows that children do best when parents can cooperate on behalf of the child. Both parents' ongoing commitment to the child's well-being is vital. If a child's symptoms become severe, see your pediatrician, and possibly a mental health professional, who can meet with the parents and child to help them learn how to make the strain of the divorce easier on the entire family.

Spending Time with Your Children

While parents may feel some guilt for not spending enough time with their children, one study shows that they are spending more time with them than parents did in the recent past. The University of Michigan study compared the amount of time parents spent in 1997 with their children with the time spent by parents in 1981. Overall, researchers found that mothers spent about four more hours a week with their children in 1997 than in 1981, and fathers spent about three hours more.

The researchers studied diaries filled out by children, ages three to twelve, and their parents that recorded how they spent their time on two days, a weekday and a weekend day. The 1981 group included 243 children, and the 1997 group included 2,125.

The biggest gains came in two-parent families. Single-parent families did not register such gains. For example, single mothers spent about twenty-one hours a week with their children in 1981 and the same number in 1997. Single mothers tend to have more restrictive work schedules at lower pay. Also, two-parent families can juggle work schedules, freeing up more time for both spouses to spend with children. For instance, fathers spend about six hours more a week with children when mothers are working.

The changes may reflect a difference in how current society sees parenting. Parents didn't feel as much pressure to spend time with their children twenty years ago. We appear to place more value on child development today. Parents have come to feel that helping their child learn and grow is important. Part of that involves spending more time together.

However, it's hard to pinpoint how, exactly, parents are spending the increased time with their children. It looks as if much of the activity is achievement oriented, such as extracurricular activities or homework. Parents seem to want to increase their children's sense of autonomy and independence. What they are less conscious of is the need for socializing and just being there.

Most important is really allowing for unstructured time with children, being aware that the parent's presence with the child is very important.

Teaching Children to Relate to People

In addition to teaching our children how to read, write, do math, and use a computer, we must teach them how to understand and relate to each other. This learning begins at home with the relationship between parent and child.

Understanding the many potential meanings of physical symptoms is crucial to the process of teaching children how to be emotionally responsive and available to others. A move by parents to teach children how to understand each other emotionally will lead to a generation of emotionally healthy children who have the basis to become emotionally healthy adults.

Ask children what they want most from their parents, and the answer is likely "to be there" when they need them and to keep up with what's happening in their lives. Parents need to establish a meaningful line of communication with their child before the difficult teen years. They should try to talk to their children in a way that prepares them for life's responsibilities. By validating the child's feelings, parents provide an invaluable opportunity to connect.

The key to communicating with children is respect. Parents need to respect their child's individuality while still maintaining their authority as parents. Some parents have difficulty accepting that the child is entitled to his or her own independent thoughts and feelings. Other parents may inadvertently try to deny children's feelings because emotions are upsetting to them. All parents need to listen with full attention and acknowledge their child's feelings.

To feel truly listened to is the basis of feeling loved. This feeling loved is part of how children form their sense of self. Listening is an important component of communication. In "What Kids Need to Succeed," a national survey of more than 100,000 children in more than 200 communities, family support and positive family communication were the two top-rated assets for successful children. Children who have these two assets are able to turn to their parents for advice and support. They are less likely to become involved with drugs, alcohol abuse, and other risk-taking behaviors. These children have frequent in-depth conversations with their parents and find their parents approachable and available.

Another way that young adolescents develop self-esteem is through religious involvement. A national survey conducted by Louisiana State University psychologists of more than 1,200 eighth graders from different parts of the United States found that those who participate in religious activities evaluate themselves more positively than those who don't participate in religious activities.

Religious activities are often something a family does together. Churches and other religious institutions teach people how to have positive images of themselves. The large influence of religious involvement on self-esteem may also infer that younger adolescents are closer with their parents, which may also play a role in their self-esteem. The relationship with parents is still strong in the younger adolescent's life, in spite of increasing importance of peer relationships. Family influence may also have an affect on an adolescent's religious involvement, which leads to more chances to receive positive teaching.

Better Parents, Happier Children

Jacob's father, Andy, brings his eight-year-old son to me for an evaluation because "he's unappreciative and just focuses on what he can get."

As examples, Andy cites Jacob's failure to thank his parents for a birthday party at an amusement park or to thank his friends for the presents. His father becomes angry at this behavior, and criticizes Jacob, which leads to prolonged fights. The fights lead Jacob to get headaches, which Andy sees as "just faking to get attention."

"When I feel something strongly, I'm not aware of anyone or anything else," says Jacob. "I'm too busy trying to hold onto my own feelings. I get the headaches when I get angry with myself, like when my team loses." I teach Jacob how to recognize some situations where he may become preoccupied with intense feelings. We talk about ways to "turn the burner down" on his feelings, which include breathing exercises, imagery, and self-talk. The imagery involves a donut-shaped block of ice that he wears like a baseball cap to "cool down" his headaches, which seems to work.

I meet with his parents and help them to communicate their concerns and expectations to Jacob without his feeling criticized. In talking with Andy, I find out that he was treated somewhat harshly by his parents, and he sees that he may be doing the same to his son. The next week, on a trip back from looking at overnight camps, Jacob thanks his parents without any prompting, causing his father to beam. Within several weeks, his headaches are gone.

Translation: "When I seem ungrateful, it's because I'm thinking about my own feelings so much I forget to say thank you."

Children basically want to be understood. Most often, difficulties between parents and children involve a misunderstanding or common communication errors. You can clear the lines so your children, and you, feel happier.

Two common errors parents make include having expectations that are not expressed to the child or that are not appropriate for the child's age. At other times, parents project their own feelings onto their children and miscalculate what their children are feeling. For example, eight-year-old Jacob might not be expected to formally thank his parents for throwing a birthday party, though his parents should try to instill in him the importance of always recognizing what other do for him, and that he should say "thanks" even if it's his parents. His parents might see he's thankful by his joyful reactions.

At other times, parents project their own feelings onto their children and miscalculate what their children are feeling. In the above example,

Andy remembers that he would not thank his parents when he was angry with them for not giving him what he really wanted. He recalled that at his Bar Mitzvah, his parents invited all of their friends and hired a band that played "their kind" of music. He did not thank his parents, knowing they expected him to, because he was quite disappointed in the party. Now he assumes Jacob's behavior has the same roots—but he is wrong, because his son is, in fact, grateful!

When parents tune into what their children are saying from early on, they build a foundation as their children grow. Being able to listen helps parents remain important figures in their children's lives. Recent research shows that adolescents lean on their parents for support even as they simultaneously push their parents away. If parents can learn to receive the messages their children send, find some common ground, and respond with warmth and love, their children will continue to listen.

To strengthen their parenting skills, parents need to get involved. Research indicates that children do better in school and have fewer behavior problems when parents are involved in their learning. In an environment of unconditional love and affection, education and learning should be stressed from an early age. Parents should establish a collaborative relationship with their children and view schoolwork as a series of projects. They should expose their children to large quantities of books. They should read to the child daily and establish an early habit of extensive and broad reading. The child's natural curiosity and sponge-like interest will take over, but parents need to jumpstart and bootstrap the process. The world of science is a wonder to all children. Parents have to introduce their children to it through books and meaningful activities, such as visits to libraries and science museums. Most importantly, parents should instill in their children a value system. Parental involvement is essential to the children's formulating an attitude and a momentum toward achieving excellence as a goal.

Parent-Child Chats Bear Repeating

When parents talk with their children about important issues, such as sex and drugs, the message doesn't always get through, at least not the first time. From one-third to more than one-half of eight- to eleven-year-olds whose parents say they have talked with them about a given issue don't remember it, according to a survey of 1,249 parents and 823 children ages eight to fifteen, which was sponsored by Children Now, an advocacy group, and Nickelodeon, the children's entertainment company. More than half of the children whose parents say they discussed HIV and AIDS don't recall the chat. To get through to children, parents should keep discussions ongoing and not make a big deal of talking once and then checking the topic off your list. Bring up sensitive topics early and often to really connect. And don't just assume if your child says he "doesn't remember" something being discussed, that it still might not be "sinking in" on a deeper level.

Action Plan

Both biological and environmental factors can cause a tendency toward violence. There are warning signs for a child's capacity to become violent, including the signs of aggression outlined earlier.

Violence doesn't just happen. It's a combination of factors—some from the child's personality, others from a lack of recognition by the child's family—that come together to make a child act violently. Just as some parents turn a blind eye to drug abuse and unsafe sex, others don't believe that their child could be aggressive or violent.

Another part of the violence problem is that many parents believe that aggression is justified. Men and boys, in particular, feel justified in reacting aggressively if they feel threatened. CDT, or "Compliance, Detection, Takedown" is a nonviolent self-defense course that is growing in popularity among adults. CDT uses nonviolent ways of subduing an attacker without physically harming him or her. CDT uses words as well as pressure points applied on the attacker's body. Community and school-based programs need to teach children in a systematic way how to deal with violence. The school's curriculum should include how to deal with aggressive feelings, sort of a diplomacy course for children. One week of studying violence in health class is not enough.

Violence with guns is not like a seizure disorder where, out of the blue, a child just snaps and starts shooting. The vast majority of children are not capable of shooting someone. They need to have a specific, underlying emotional pattern and be subjected to the right amount of stress and violence.

When it comes to school shootings, the schools and parents have reacted with their own agendas. They sometimes say it could not be predicted, that the shooter was a nice boy with no problems. If he was on medication, then the drug is the problem, not the child, they sometimes claim. However, if the shooting has nothing to do with anything within our control as parents and educators, then we might as well throw our hands up and give up. In these shootings, it is not psychiatric medication that is causing the children to pull the trigger.

We can educate people and train them to predict and prevent potential disasters. You can learn to identify which children are predisposed to violence through workshops in the community and at school. I believe that educators should take a regular course on violence. These school programs should describe how to handle violence with an emotionally based approach, which is what now happens for drug abuse. Some states are now instituting such programs about violence and guns for school children.

The main issue with guns is access. The data are clear about one thing—the more guns that are available, the more people get shot. I agree with the American Academy of Pediatrics' recommendation that the safest way to avoid a firearm injury in the home is to remove guns from the home. Parents should also ask about the presence of guns in places where their children play or visit.

In principle, zero tolerance about violence is reasonable, but many schools are more worried about covering themselves legally than really helping children. The school has to go beyond simply looking for red flags and barring problem students from school. We need school-based programs that deal with problem resolution, not simply sending students to hear a lecture about violence.

Conflict is inescapable, and that's why conflict resolution programs are essential. Parents can help children with conflict resolution. Instead of telling your child "If he bothers you again, whack him," come up with ways together to resolve the conflict with nonviolent means. I recommend that parents read everything they can get their hands on about youth violence. The Surgeon General's Report on

Violence is good place to start. This report called for a commission to look at this issue, which I heartily agree with.

Some amount of violence will always be in our world, no matter what. We can address and control it to some extent, as we do crime. Violence will continue to be a problem until parents do something about it. Pay more attention to what your children are doing. Become more aware of what sites your child is visiting on the Internet, what music she listens to, and what movies she sees. Take an active role early on in discussing how violence is not an acceptable first response. As your child gets older, maintain some degree of vigilance. This has to be a long-term, multi-pronged approach.

For tragic events, such as war or terrorism, you can help your child cope. A preschooler may hear about a disaster from television or older children, but don't bring the tragedy to your child's attention unless you know he or she is aware of it. Use this moment as an opportunity to teach how to express emotions, including anger, in a healthy way. A young child feels more comfortable knowing a parent is near. Show your child things that keep your family safe, such as the alarm system or door locks. Younger children may have trouble expressing themselves with words, so offer to draw together, and then discuss the feelings depicted in the pictures.

Older children may know the news through television or friends. Ask what your child really knows, and go from there. The answer should give you a clue about what's on your child's mind. Discuss what you can do as a family to make your community safer. If your child is afraid, don't dismiss the feelings. Comfort and let your child know that you are there and that you will work through this together.

You may become preoccupied, anxious, and sad by a disaster, but you must guard against showing your children that you are so afraid. Realize that your own anxiety is contagious, so try not to let your child know that you're really nervous. Live life as normally as possible. Use your natural supports and talk with those you feel comfortable with—friends, family, coworkers—at your own pace. And don't become too glued to the tube and unavailable to your children when they need you the most. You may find more advice and helpful tips from Internet chat rooms and bulletin boards. There, you can connect with other parents who may be going through a similar difficulty.

Traumatic experiences may stir up memories or exacerbate symptoms related to previous traumatic events. You may feel as if old wounds have opened up again. These symptoms will likely abate with time. It may be helpful to remember what strategies you have used successfully in the past to deal with this situation, and to continue to use them. If not, you should seek some professional help.

Children are suggestible and easily over-stimulated. You can help by monitoring and controlling the amount of violence they are exposed to through television and the Internet. From a young age, your child's time is filled up with things you help them discover. Children who get involved in violence often have a lot of free time on their hands. They usually are not athletes or artists. Those who take pride in what they do are more likely to stay out of trouble.

Not every child is an athlete or an artist. They can do other things—play a musical instrument, participate in after-school activities, volunteer or work at your church or synagogue. It's important for you as a parent to help your child develop an interest at an early age. This activity provides a focus and something your child can take pride in and carry through into adolescence. It also helps to have a social network, to be around other people who also are committed to maintaining a high level at whatever your child chooses to do.

The extent of your child's commitment will depend somewhat on his or her health, both mentally and physically. You can help your child have a sense of balance between work and play. Even if a child is a talented computer programmer, spending ten hours a day at the computer probably is not healthy, mentally or physically. Such a child may be socially distanced because he spends so much time alone, plus that much computer time is not good for a child's posture or the eyes. Look at the domains described earlier in this book, including your child's involvement with school, friends, and family. An assessment of your child's life will give you an overall sense of proportion. If your child is a little shy, she should still go out with friends. Even if your son is not athletic, he should get some exercise. For teens, make sure they eat right and have reasonable sleep habits.

Parents can shape their children's lifestyles from an early age, which involves diet, rest, exercise, creative outlets, quality time with parents, and how to apportion time for both work and play. When it comes to diet and exercise, try not to talk out of both sides of your mouth. If you lead a healthy lifestyle, and your children see you exercising or playing sports, they are more likely to do that. Parent by example. A child's formative years are important for establishing consistent values, resolving conflicts, and getting involved in activities.

Decisions on food start in the home. Parents have to think of themselves as their child's advocates. As a parent, you walk a fine line between making food an emotional issue that gets ingrained in childhood versus trying to help your child have great self-esteem and be proud. But you can only go so far. At some point, your child will have to take control of food problems.

It's often counterproductive to get into a power struggle with your child about food. Encouraging your child to diet may result in his or her weight yo-yoing up and down. Instead, stop being a "food cop" and start becoming more actively involved as a family with what your child eats, how the food is prepared, and how much everybody exercises together. These changes can also reduce your child's stress. I suggest that you intervene when your child's weight is diverging upward from a normal growth curve. Ask your pediatrician for help in looking at this trend.

Emphasize physical activity to help reduce weight. Exercise means you will have to do more than say, "Go outside and play." To get your child moving, you may need to take a bike ride or hike together. Any kind of movement and play can be fun. Turn on some music and dance, go out and toss a Frisbee, or play ball; do anything your child would enjoy.

Parents and children can find tips for healthy eating and incorporating exercise into their day on a Web page produced by the President's Council on Physical Fitness and Sports (*www.fitness.gov/funfit/funfit.html*). The government also provides a Food Guide Pyramid site for toddlers and children, ages two to six, on the Web at (*www.usda.gov/news/usdakids/food_pyr.html*).

Children older than six can use the regular Food Guide Pyramid chart (*www.nal.usda.gov/fnic/Fpyr/pyramid.html*). The President's Council Web site also has ways to motivate your child in *Get Fit! A Handbook for Youth Ages 6–17*. KidsHealth (*www.kidshealth.com*) is a comprehensive medical site that answers children's questions in simple language on such issues as being too fat or too thin, is dieting okay, and how to stay fit even if you don't like sports.

Spend time with your children and do leisure activities that your child chooses. As I've indicated, children can become stressed from overscheduling activities. I believe it's better for a child to have his eggs in only a few baskets, and invest some time and effort with a teacher's aid. Then you're more likely to see some good returns. If your child has too many eggs in too many baskets, then the child may not establish some competency or proficiency.

Sometimes you have to decide what is best for your child. It's like eating vegetables. We all want our children to eat right, including their vegetables. How far you push is a matter of finesse and priorities. If your daughter likes to read novels, get her into something social, such as Brownies, or a physical activity. I think all children should have the opportunity to explore their own capabilities. That's why I require my children to do extracurricular activities, from taking piano lessons to taking up sports such as soccer, tennis, and karate.

Straightforward talk with your children about drugs is essential. Start from the time they are young so this is not a new topic you've never brought up before they become teens. If your child goes to parties, find out what people are drinking and smoking. Encourage them to be honest. If they say they are tempted to try something, look at this as an opening to discuss the situation. If you immediately forbid your child from seeing these friends or attending parties, she may never open up to you again. Use things in media, for example, television commercials about the dangers of drug abuse, as an easy way to bring up drugs.

Drug abuse prevention is similar to prevention of other high-risk behaviors. Children with a family history of substance abuse, impulsive behavior, and social difficulties may be at high risk of drug abuse. Most teens experiment with drugs to "be cool." Early identification of those at risk or who use drugs is important. If you are suspicious about drug abuse, have your child tested for drugs with your pediatrician's help. If the child tests positive for drugs and is a regular drug user, get him or her into a treatment program.

It's important to communicate openly about sexuality. Parents can't abdicate their responsibilities. If you don't know how to talk to your children about sex, or feel uncomfortable about it, get some help from a physician, guidance counselor, psychologist, or someone who has experience talking to teens. STDs can be prevented with sex education. Discussions about STDs with sexually active teens should include questions about theirs access to condoms. STDs are generally underreported among teens, who are not that honest about whether they have had an STD.

But avoiding STDs is not the only sex education issue. Health education programs to prevent teen pregnancy have been tried, with varied success, but we have to keep trying. You can't just ignore the issue and think others will take care of it. In particular, don't ignore a child who asks for birth control. Any teen who asks for help about birth control should get it, as well as counseling from a doctor, guidance counselor, psychologist, or psychiatrist. You want to combine talking about birth control with making sure your teen has safe sex. Studies show that use of condoms can reduce STDs.

Limit your kids "screen" time, whether it's computers, television, or hand-held video games. While these activities help children deal well with boredom, they are a form of self-stimulation and avoidance. I'd rather have a bored child call a friend or go outside and run around. My children are allowed to watch one hour of television a day on weekdays, and two hours a day on weekends.

Teens like to cybersurf for health and other types of information. Some of that is good. Studies show that cognitive behavior therapy provided online can help conquer eating disorders. Chat rooms are double-edged swords. They allow children to talk to friends, blow off steam, or find others with similar problems or similar illnesses, such as cystic fibrosis. Used as a local social network, the Internet can be fine. But you have to know what's going on in chat rooms. Children can get a lot of misinformation from them. Plus there's the risk for online sex solicitation. Many young people who use the Internet have to counter unwanted sexual overtures. You should encourage your child to report any solicitation of sex to you. You may have gone over what to do if a stranger comes up to your children on the street, but they need to know how to handle strangers on the computer too. Some socially anxious or lonely teens cultivate "virtual" relationships on the Internet instead of "real" relationships. These relationships can become quite obsessive and take up large amounts of a teen's time, or keep him or her up to all hours of the night. Sometimes, this can lead to "real" encounters if the parties decide to meet, which may involve extensive travel, and rarely work out positively.

When it comes to the media, look for literature that's age appropriate, and make time to read with your child, or have your child read to you, before you turn on the television. Children are faced with violence everywhere in the media, even in so-called *E*-rated video games. Before you let your child play a video game, play it yourself, just as you would screen a book or a movie before your child read or watched it.

For single parents, I suggest they find help with other role models or relatives that can influence their child's life. Besides aunts, uncles, and family friends, some single parents may qualify for other resources, such as a visiting nurse. If need be, place your child in an after-school program, where he or she will be supervised. Remember, children learn by example, so single parents who are dating need to pay close attention to their own behavior, in particular regarding having a date sleep over. The challenge may be greater for single parents, but they need to make similar attempts to spend quality time with their children.

The main message I've tried to give in this book is: Understand your child and establish a close relationship early on, then keep the lines of communication open. Children want to listen and understand at an early age. When they get older, and may not want to talk, you still need to oversee what they are doing and with whom they associate. Teens walk a fine line between independence and autonomy and supervision. Teach good values early on, by the examples you set or through your religious organization. Have a strong sense of family values. Most children who get into trouble with violence have problems with self-esteem. Throughout this book the emphasis has been on raising your child's self-esteem. Safeguard it to ensure that it grows.

Tell Me Where It Hurts begins with the physical, a child who has tummyaches or headaches, and perhaps is sad or nervous. On a more philosophical scale, this request is a call for parents to understand the stresses, challenges, and pain that their children may experience as they grow up. If we, as parents, can help our children keep the lines of communication open, we can continue to give them our guidance, love, encouragement, and acceptance, and help them grow safely into happy adults.

Action Points

1. Know the warning signs of aggression that may lead to violence.
2. If you have a gun, keep it locked safely away from your child. Ask about guns in the homes of your child's friends.
3. Use war or terrorism as a "teachable moment" to better understand how to express feelings. Don't dismiss your child's fearful or angry feelings.
4. Control exposure to violence through computers, television, and the media.
5. Help shape your child's lifestyle, and provide a healthy example.
6. Get active with your child. Do something he or she wants to do with you.
7. Begin discussing drugs when your child is young to make it easier to talk about it when he or she reaches teenage.
8. Talk openly about sex and STDs, and make sure your child is practicing safe sex.
9. Limit your child's "screen time" with television, computers, and hand-held games.
10. Know which Web sites your child is visiting and video games he or she is playing.
11. Single parents need to find help through relatives or other role models.
12. Establish a close relationship with your child to help safeguard his or her self-esteem.

Resources

Books

Recommended resources for information on psychotropic medications for children:

Timothy E. Wilens, M.D., (1999), *Straight Talk about Psychiatric Medications for Kids*. The Guilford Press, *www.guilford.com*.

Mina K. Dulcan and Tami Benton (1999), *Helping Parents, Youth, and Teachers Understand Medications for Behavioral and Emotional Problems: A Resource Book of Medication Information Handouts*. American Psychiatric Press, Washington, DC.

John Scott Werry, M.D., and Michal G. Aman, Ph.D., (1999), *Practitioner's Guide to Psychoactive Drugs for Children and Adolescents*. 2nd edition. Kluwer Academic/Plenum Publishers, New York, NY.

Recommended reading about stress:

Robert M. Zapolsky, (1998), *Why Zebras Don't Get Ulcers*. W. H. Freeman and Company. New York, NY.

Michael D. Gershon, M.D., (1998), *The Second Brain*. HarperCollins Publishers, New York, NY.

Web Sites

www.jonathanslater.com
www.ncbi.nlm.nih.gov/entrez/query.fcgi
www.medem.com
www.mentalhealth.com
www.aacap.org
www.nimh.nih.gov

User-friendly Web sites for several classes of medications and supplements used in the treatment of bipolar disorder include:

Atypical neuroleptics
www.bipolarchild.com/newsletters/0010.html
Mood stabilizers
www.bipolarchild.com/newsletters/0003.html
www.bpkids.org/learning/about.htm
Omega-3 fatty acids
www.bipolarchild.com/newsletters/0501.html

References from professional literature, with links

www.bpkids.org/learning/references.htm

Organizations

American Academy of Child and Adolescent Psychiatry
3615 Wisconsin Ave., N.W.
Washington, DC 20016-3007
Phone: 202-966-7300
Fax: 202-966-2891
Web site: *www.aacap.org*

American Academy of Sleep Medicine
6301 Bandel Rd., #101
Rochester, MN 55901
Phone: 507-287-6006
Fax: 507-287-6008
Web site: *www.aasmnet.org*
E-mail: *info@aasmnet.org*

American Chronic Pain Association
P.O. Box 850
Rocklin, CA 95677
Phone: 916-632-0922
Fax: 916-632-3208
Web site: *www.theacpa.org*
E-mail: *acpa@pacbell.net*

Anxiety Disorders Association of America
11900 Parklawn Dr., Suite 100
Rockville, MD 20852-2624
Phone: 301-231-9350
Fax: 301-231-7392
Web site: *www.adaa.org*
E-mail: *anxdis@aol.com*

Autism Society of America
7910 Woodmont Ave., Suite 300
Bethesda, MD 20814-3015
Phone: 800-328-8476
Fax: 301-657-0869
Web site: *www.autism-society.org*

Children and Adults with Attention Deficit Disorders (CH.A.D.D.)
8181 Professional Pl., Suite 201
Landover, MD 20785
Phone: 800-233-4050
Fax: 301-306-7090
Web site: *www.chadd.org*
E-mail: *national@chadd.org*

Juvenile Bipolar Research Foundation
49 South Quaker Hill Road
Pawling, NY 12564
Phone: 203-226-2216
Web site: *www.bpchildresearch.org*

Learning Disabilities Association of America
4156 Library Rd.
Pittsburgh, PA 15234
Phone: 888-300-6710
Fax: 412-344-0224
Web site: *www.ldaamerica.org*
E-mail: *idanatl@usaor.net*

National Alliance for Research on Schizophrenia and Depression
60 Cutter Mill Rd., Suite 404
Great Neck, NY 11021
Phone: 800-829-8289
Fax: 516-487-6930
Web site: *www.narsad.org*

National Association of Anorexia Nervosa and Associated Disorders
P.O. Box 7
Highland Park, IL 60035
Phone: 847-831-3438
Fax: 847-433-4632
Web site: *www.anad.org*
E-mail: *anad20@aol.com*

National Center for Complementary and Alternative Medicine Information Clearinghouse
P.O. Box 8218
Silver Spring, MD 20907-8218
Phone: 888-644-6226
Fax: 301-495-4957
Web site: *www.nih.gov*
E-mail: *nccam-info@nccam.nih.gov*

National Depressive and Manic-Depressive Association
730 N. Franklin, #501
Chicago, IL 60610
Phone: 800-826-3632
Fax: 312-642-7243
Web site: *www.ndmda.org*
E-mail: *myrtis@aol.com*

National Headache Foundation
428 W. St. James Pl., 2nd Fl.
Chicago, IL 60614-2710
Phone: 888-643-5552
Fax: 773-525-7357
Web site: *www.headaches.org*
E-mail: *info@headaches.org*

National Institute of Mental Health Public Inquiries
6001 Executive Boulevard, Rm. 8184, MSC 9663
Bethesda, MD 20092-9663
Phone: 301-443-4513
Fax: 301-443-4279
Web site: *www.nimh.nih.gov*
E-mail: *nimhinfo@nih.gov*

Obsessive-Compulsive Foundation (OCD)
337 Notch Hill Rd.
North Branford, CT 06471
Phone: 203-315-2190
Fax: 203-315-2196
Web site: *www.ocfoundation.org*
E-mail: *info@ocfoundation.org*

Tourette Syndrome Association
42–40 Bell Blvd.
Bayside, NY 11361
Phone: 800-237-0717
Fax: 718-279-9596
Web site: *www.tsa-usa.org*
E-mail: *tourette@ix.netcom.com*

References

Bahrke, MS, Yesalis, CE, and Brower, KJ. "Anabolic-androgenic steroid abuse and performance-enhancing drugs among adolescents." *Child Adoles. Psych.* Clinics of NA 1998 Oct; 7 (4):821–38.

Baker, J, et. al. "The relationship between coaching behaviours and sport anxiety in athletes." *J Sci Med Sport* 2000 Jun; 3 (2):110–19.

Burd L, et. al. "Long-term follow-up of an epidemiologically defined cohort of patients with Tourette syndrome." *J Child Neurol* 2001 Jun; 16 (6):431–7.

Campbell, M. "Antipsychotics in Children and Adolescents." *J Am Acad Child Adoles Psychiatry* 1999; 38:537–545.

Coplan, JD, et. al. "Persistent elevations of cerebrospinal fluid concentrations of corticotropin-releasing factor in adult nonhuman primates exposed to early-life stressors: implications for the pathophysiology of mood and anxiety disorders." *Proc Natl Acad Sci* 1996 Feb 20; 93 (4):1619–23.

Donovan, SJ, et. al. "Divalproex treatment of disruptive adolescents: a report of 10 cases." *J Clin Psychiatry* 1997 Jan; 58 (1):12–15.

Egger, HL, et. al. "Somatic complaints and psychopathology in children and adolescents: stomachaches, musculoskeletal pains, and headaches." *J Am Acad Child Adolesc Psychiatry* 1999 Jul; 38 (7):852–60.

Emslie, GJ, et. al. "A double-blind, randomized, placebo controlled trial of fluoxetine in children and adolescents with depression." *Arch Gen Psychiatry* 1997 Nov; 54 (11)1031–37.

Emslie, GJ, et. al. "Nontricyclic Antidepressants Current Trends in Children and Adolescents." *J Am Acad Child Adoles Psychiatry* 1999; 38:517–528.

Fahlke, C, et. al. "Rearing experiences and stress-induced plasma cortisol as early risk factors for excessive alcohol consumption in nonhuman primates." *Alcohol Clin Exp Res* 2000 May; 24 (5):644–50.

Ford, IW, et. al. "An examination of psychosocial variables moderating the relationship between life stress and injury time-loss among athletes of a high standard." *J Sports Sci* 2000 May; 18 (5):301–12.

Geller, B, et. al. "Critical Review of Tricyclic Antidepressant Use in Children and Adolescents." *J Am Acad Child Adoles Psychiatry* 1999; 38:513–516.

Greenhill, LL, et. al. "Stimulant Medications." *J Am Acad Child Adoles Psychiatry* 1999; 38:503–512.

Herman-Toffler, LR, et. al. "The effects of aerobic training on children's creativity, self-perception, and aerobic power." *Child Adoles. Psych. Clinics of NA* 1998 Oct; 7 (4):773–90.

Jensen, PS, et. al. "Findings from the NIMH Multimodal Treatment Study of ADHD (MTA): implications and applications for primary care providers." *J Dev Behav Pediatr* 2001 Feb; 22 (1):60–73.

Kamm, RL. "A developmental and psychoeducational approach to reducing conflict and abuse in Little League and youth sports: The Sport Psychiatrist's Role." *Child Adoles. Psych.* Clinics of NA 1998 Oct; 7 (4):891–918.

Keller, MB, et. al. "Efficacy of paroxetine in the treatment of adolescent major depression: a randomized, controlled trial." *J Am Acad Child Adoles Psychiatry* 2001 July; 40 (7):762–72.

Kendall, PC, et. al. "Comorbidity in childhood anxiety disorders and treatment outcome." *J Am Acad Child Adoles Psychiatry* 2001 July; 40 (7):787–94.

Kessler, RC. "Long-term trends in the use of complementary and alternative medical therapies in the United States." *Annals of Internal Medicine* 2001 August 21; 135(4):262–268.

Kiecolt-Glaser, JK, et.al. "Psychoneuroimmunology and psychosomatic medicine: back to the future." *Psychosom Med* 2002 Jan–Feb; 64 (1):15–28.

Kuperman, S, et. al. "Relationship of child psychopathology to parental alcoholism and antisocial personality disorder." *J Am Acad Child Adoles Psychiatry* 1999 June; 38 (6):686–92.

Kowatch, RA, et. al. "Effect size of lithium, divalproex sodium, and carbamazepine in children and adolescents with bipolar disorder." *J Am Acad Child Adolesc Psychiatry* 2000 Jun; 39 (6):713–20.

Leckman, JF, et. al. "Course of tic severity in Tourette syndrome: the first two decades." *Pediatrics* 1998 Jul; 102 (1 Pt 1):14–9.

Levy, RL, et. al. "Family stress and behavior problems are associated with more gastrointestinal symptoms and school absences." May 22, 2001. Presentation at Digestive Disease Week annual meeting.

Libman, S. "Adult participation in youth sports: A developmental perspective." *Child Adoles. Psych. Clinics of NA* 1998 Oct; 7 (4):725–44.

Muris, P, et. al. "Worry in normal children." *J. Am. Acad. Child Adolesc. Psychiatry* 1998; 37 (7):703–710.

Nansel, TR, et. al. "Bullying behaviors among US youth." *JAMA* 2001 April 25; 285 (16):2094–2100.

Nicholson, R, et. al. "Children and adolescents with psychotic disorder not otherwise specified: a 2- to 8-year follow-up study." *Compr Psychiatry* 2001 Jul–Aug; 42 (4):319–25.

Olness, K, et. al. "Voluntary regulation of salivary immunoglobulin A." *Pediatrics* 1988; 1989 Jan; 83 (1):66–71.

Quas, JA, et. al. "Dissociations between psychobiologic reactivity and emotional expression in children." *Dev Psychobiol* 2000 Nov; 37 (3):153–75.

Riddle, MA, et. al. "Anxiolytics, Adrenergic Agents, and Naltrexone" *J Am Acad Child & Adoles Psychiatry* 1999; 38:546–556.

Ryan, ND, et. al. "Mood Stabilizers in Children and Adolescents." *J Am Acad Child Adoles Psychiatry* 1999; 38:529–536.

Spiegel, D, et.al. "Supportive-expressive group therapy and life extension of breast cancer patients: Spiegel et al. (1989)" *Advance in Mind-Body Medicine* 2001;17:38-41.

Stryer, BK, et. al. "A developmental overview of child and youth sports in society." *Child Adoles. Psych.* Clinics of NA 1998 Oct; 7 (4):697–724.

The Research Unit on Pediatric Psychopharmacology Anxiety Study Group. "Fluvoxamine for the treatment of anxiety disorders in children and adolescents: The Research Unit on Pediatric Psychopharmacology Anxiety Study Group." *N Engl J Med* 2001 Apr 26; 344 (17):1279-85.

Thompson, KM, and Haninger, K. "Violence in e-rated video games." JAMA 2001 August 1; 286 (5):591–98.

Villani, S. "Impact of media on children and adolescents: a 10-year review of the research." *J. Am. Acad. Child Adolesc. Psychiatry* 2001 April; 40 (4):392–400.

Whitehead, WE, et. al. "Children's gastrointestinal complaints and family size." May 22, 2001. Presentation at Digestive Disease Week annual meeting.

Zito JM, et. al. "Trends in the prescribing of psychotropic medications to preschoolers." *JAMA* 2000 Feb 23; 283 (8):1059–60.

Zuddas A, et. al. "Long-term risperidone for pervasive developmental disorder: efficacy, tolerability, and discontinuation." *J Child Adolesc Psychopharmacol* Summer 2000; 10 (2):79–90.

Index

About the Authors

Jonathan Slater, M.D., graduated from Harvard University and received his medical doctorate from Columbia University. He did postgraduate research at the New York Psychiatric Institute, studying the pharmacological treatment of aggression. He completed both an adult psychiatric residency and child/adolescent psychiatry fellowship at the New York State Psychiatric Institute. He was certified in psychoanalysis by the Columbia University Center for Psychoanalytic Training and Research.

Board certified in adult psychiatry and child and adolescent psychiatry, Dr. Slater is the Chief of Pediatric Psychiatry Consultation-Liaison at Children's Hospital of New York, part of New York–Presbyterian Medical Center, and is an Associate Professor of Psychiatry at Columbia University. In addition, he is the Attending Psychiatrist for the Pediatric Cardiac Transplant team.

Dr. Slater's research interests include a recent investigation using circus clowns to decrease psychological distress in children undergoing invasive medical procedures. He has published chapters in four medical books about such topics as child development, psychopharmacology in medically ill children, and the psychological effects of transplantation and cancer on children. Dr. Slater has received four medical awards for his clinical work from the Psychiatric Institute, and a teaching award from Columbia University's medical school for the Child Development course he teaches to medical students. Dr. Slater worked as a consultant and contributing producer on an HBO documentary film, *Heart of a Child*. He also completed a two-hour documentary video, *Second Chance: Heroes of Heart Transplantation in Children*.

Dr. Slater is a Black Belt in karate who trains and teaches at the New York Goju Karate Association in Hastings-on-Hudson, New York, where he lives with his wife and four children.

Health and medical writer Mark L. Fuerst is the coauthor of six books, including *Sports Injury Handbook* (John Wiley) and *The Couple's Guide to Fertility* (Broadway Books), now in its third edition. As a freelance journalist for twenty-five years, his articles have appeared in popular consumer magazines such as *Family Circle*, *Woman's Day*, and *Health*. His articles on children's health have appeared in *American Health*, *Self*, *Good Housekeeping*, *Parents*, and various newspaper syndicates.

Mr. Fuerst earned a biology degree from Dickinson College and a master's degree in journalism from the University of Missouri at Columbia. He has been a member of the National Association of Science Writers for more than two dozen years and a member of the American Society of Journalists and Authors for more than twenty years, for which he served as president from 1992 to 1994. He lives in Brooklyn, NY, with his wife and two children.